PRACTI... ...H
OLDER

...s due for return on or before the last date shown below.

FORTHCOMING TITLES

Occupational Therapy for the Brain-Injured Adult
Jo Clark-Wilson and Gordon Muir Giles

Multiple Sclerosis
Approaches to management
Lorraine De Souza

Modern Electrotherapy
Mary Dyson and Christopher Hayne

Autism
A multidisciplinary approach
Edited by Kathryn Ellis

Physiotherapy in Respiratory and Intensive Care
Alexandra Hough

Community Occupational Therapy with Mentally Handicapped People
Debbie Isaac

Understanding Dysphasia
Lesley Jordan and Rita Twiston Davies

Management in Occupational Therapy
Zielfa B. Maslin

Dysarthria
Theory and therapy
Sandra J. Robertson

Speech and Language Problems in Children
Dilys A. Treharne

THERAPY IN PRACTICE SERIES

Edited by Jo Campling

This series of books is aimed at 'therapists' concerned with rehabilitation in a very broad sense. The intended audience particularly includes occupational therapists, physiotherapists and speech therapists, but many titles will also be of interest to nurses, psychologists, medical staff, social workers, teachers or volunteer workers. Some volumes will be interdisciplinary, others aimed at one particular profession. All titles will be comprehensive but concise, and practical but with due reference to relevant theory and evidence. They are not research monographs but focus on professional practice, and will be of value to both students and qualified personnel.

1. Occupational Therapy for Children with Disabilities
   Dorothy E. Penso
2. Living Skills for Mentally Handicapped People
   Christine Peck and Chia Swee Hong
3. Rehabilitation of the Older Patient
   Edited by Amanda J. Squires
4. Physiotherapy and the Elderly Patient
   Paul Wagstaff and Davis Coakley
5. Rehabilitation of the Severely Brain-Injured Adult
   Edited by Ian Fussey and Gordon Muir Giles
6. Communication Problems in Elderly People
   Rosemary Gravell
7. Occupational Therapy Practice in Psychiatry
   Linda Finlay
8. Working with Bilingual Language Disability
   Edited by Deirdre M. Duncan
9. Counselling Skills for Health Professionals
   Philip Burnard
10. Teaching Interpersonal Skills
    A handbook of experiential learning for health professionals
    Philip Burnard
11. Occupational Therapy for Stroke Rehabilitation
    Simon Thompson and Mary Anne Morgan
12. Assessing Physically Disabled People at Home
    Kathleen Maczka
13. Acute Head Injury
    Practical management in rehabilitation
    Ruth Garner
14. Practical Physiotherapy with Older People
    Lucinda Smyth et al.
15. Keyboard, Graphic and Handwriting Skills
    Helping people with motor disabilities
    Dorothy E. Penso

Practical Physiotherapy with Older People

LUCINDA SMYTH

With contributions by
Rowena Kinsman
Helen Ransome
and Patricia Smith

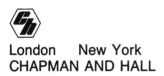

London   New York
CHAPMAN AND HALL

First published in 1990 by
Chapman and Hall Ltd
11 New Fetter Lane, London EC4P 4EE

© 1990 Chapman and Hall

Typeset in 10/12 Times by
Mayhew Typesetting, Bristol
Printed in Great Britain by
St. Edmundsbury Press, Bury St. Edmunds, Suffolk

ISBN 0 412 33580 8

British Library Cataloguing in Publication Data

Smyth, Lucinda
  Practical physiotherapy with older people.
  1. Old persons. Physiotherapy
  I. Title
  615.8′2
  ISBN 0–412–33580–8

Contents

Contributors

Rowena Kinsman
District Physiotherapist
Barnet Health Authority, London

Helen Ransome
District Physiotherapist
Lewisham and North Southwark Health Authority, London

Patricia Smith
Senior Physiotherapist
Barnet Health Authority, London

Lucinda Smyth
Community Physiotherapist
Norwich Health Authority, Norwich

Acknowledgements

The author would like to thank the contributors for their chapters in this book. In the preparation of the first four chapters valuable help was provided by physiotherapists' advice especially Lorna Cushnie, and the librarian Stephanie Skene of the Norfolk and Norwich Institute for Medical Education. Thanks are due to the Trustees of the Bicentenary Trust of this Institute for financial support. For encouragement and painstaking word processing sincere gratitude is offered to Muriel West.

Preface

Contrary to popular belief, practice of physiotherapy with elderly patients is no easy option. In addition to grappling with the effects of multipathology it presents problems of accommodating to the patients' altering physiological state and the accumulating life events of older age. There are challenges of ethics in decision making. In therapeutic management it is sometimes hard to know where to begin, what to try, and when to stop or offer something else. The work offers both satisfaction and despair, frustration and enormous interest.

Despite the existence of many specialist textbooks on medicine and physiotherapy, it is widely felt there is a place for a basic guide to physiotherapy with elderly people. This book aims to provide guidance and insights based on the writers' experience, as well as from the current literature. Good practice must be holistic in its breadth of knowledge and attitude to the individual, but meticulous in attention to detail in examination and treatment as for a patient of any age.

The key points of good practice described in this book have been validated. In order to devise a syllabus for physiotherapists studying this specialty, twelve experienced physiotherapists prepared separately lists of what each considered to be the 'key' points in good practice. These were found to be almost identical. An audit was conducted among the membership of the then Association of Chartered Physiotherapists in Geriatric Medicine (120 physiotherapists). The 80% return confirmed the importance of these key points. The Association prepared a small booklet based on this advice, and 2000 copies have been sold to physiotherapists and other health professionals. Informal canvassing of opinion has confirmed that this booklet if enlarged would provide a useful handbook on physiotherapy with older people. This book is the result. The Association, now called the Association of Chartered Physiotherapists with a Special Interest in Elderly People, is the informal sponsor of this project.

Each of the seven 'key' points in good practice becomes the topic for a chapter. Definition of each point of physiotherapy practice is followed by a description. The final part of each chapter attempts to summarize how this part of the practice differs with respect to older as compared to younger people. The first four chapters deal with physiotherapy and the patient as an individual, the next two are about relationships with other health professionals and health maintenance, and the last is on quality of care with advice to the physiotherapist on its achievement. In Chapters four and seven the sections 'Where do I begin' and 'How do I continue', describe activity in sequence, the second being based on the first. The last chapter not only describes accepted current methods but projects forward in describing new concepts which are only just beginning in practice. The order of chapters does not imply a fixed sequence or level of importance, but each informs the others. Common concepts and activities are repeated and used throughout the book and in patient care. For example, examination and evaluation should take place repeatedly. The subject matter covers a broad span, some parts being more applicable to individual physiotherapists than others. Many subjects in a book of this scope can only be introduced. Suggestions of material for further reading is provided in the bibliography for those who wish to pursue subjects in greater depth.

Although the term 'elderly' in this book is used (according to convention) as a universal label for people aged over 65 years, they do not, of course, conform to a type. No one would assume that a group of people aged between 35 and 65 would be homogeneous except in superficial ways. To an even greater extent due to physical, psychological and social factors, the range of difference among people between 65 and 95 or upward, must be wider.

The majority of very elderly patients encountered by physiotherapists are female. At present most therapists are female. Nevertheless, unless stated otherwise, the patient is usually referred to as male and the therapist as female for reasons of clarity and convenience.

The aim in producing this book is to promote good quality care and to engender in other physiotherapists as much enthusiasm for this area of work as the authors have enjoyed.

Lucinda Smyth

xii

1

Examination and assessment

Good physiotherapy practice requires an accurate examination, assessment and recording of each patient's physical state, taking into account individual psychosocial and environmental needs. This must be followed by continued re-assessment and review.

WHY EXAMINE?

The purpose of examination is to obtain a knowledge of the patient in order to assess whether he could be helped by a physiotherapy intervention and, if so, in which of his difficulties and in what manner. It involves investigation of all appropriate signs and symptoms with some historical and social background. The manner of this initial encounter sets the tone of the relationship between physiotherapist and patient which is of great importance for the outcome of the subsequent decisions.

People are referred to a physiotherapist for a variety of reasons. It may be a request for an opinion on the likelihood of success and expected time scale to achieve a certain outcome, or advice to the referrer on possible reasons for a patient's apparent immobility. Frequently, there is a plain request for intervention, relief of symptoms, and restoration of activity. If the patient is in hospital the initial reason for admission will usually have been for diagnosis, surgery or medical treatment. A possible need for physiotherapy may be identified thereafter but not necessarily connected with the problem on admission

Example: Mr Hutson, an elderly man, had been admitted for a prostatectomy. The operation has been successful so he should be

1

ready to go home so far as the surgeon is concerned. However, the nurses report that he cannot walk and is reluctant to help himself. He is referred to the physiotherapist to be 'mobilized'.

In the community, patients are commonly referred via the general practitioner if treatment, or a professional opinion is requested. There are occasions when advice is sought by social service employees or a nurse. Care assistants in a residential home might be noticing increasing difficulty in helping a disabled person on to the toilet, and ask either for advice on alternative methods or that the resident's strength be improved. A district nurse might ask whether her patient's balance might be more secure using a walking aid.

The focus of physiotherapy interest and treatment is not always what the general practitioner sees.

Example: Mrs Jewson, living with her daughter complains to her doctor of dizziness and falls. He finds slight signs and symptoms in the cardiovascular system that need medical care. In order to prevent further falls the physiotherapist is asked to provide a walking frame. During examination she finds additionally that the patient's knee joints and one of her wrists are stiff and painful. This has made climbing stairs very difficult and this is the site where one fall has occurred.

Both these patients could be presenting rehabilitation problems of considerable complexity. In both cases, the reason for admission to hospital or consulting the doctor could be quite different from the reason to see a physiotherapist. In both cases it would be unwise to expect their problems to be single or the unravelling simple.

To jump to conclusions and assume the mobility problems could be solved by the provision of a walking frame might seem the obvious short cut. Examination of both patients, however, could reveal clinical information and problems of which the referrer was unaware, but which are of importance to the physiotherapist's management of that situation.

Example: Mr Hutson on examination may be found to be confused due to the residual effects of anaesthetic or carbon dioxide retention due to chronic airways disease but which at first sight had seemed like a lack of willingness to co-operate. He may just have failed to put his hearing aid firmly in place. His difficulty in moving might be due to the effect of osteoarthrosis and bed rest, the stiffness induced by a previous slight hemiparesis or Parkinson's disease. Awareness of such features will alter the physiotherapist's approach and manner of treatment.

2

Example: Mrs Jewson's usual level of activity could have been affected, not by any physical change in her knees directly, but an upset or a bereavement or change of dwelling to one with more or steeper stairs. Her ascent may have been dependent on using both hands to pull herself up, but one had been painful recently and given way, causing her to lose hold on the bannister. It may be that the daughter's failing health or strength has diminished the amount of help that had been provided. Signs found by the general practitioner were only a part of her story.

In neither of these cases had the cause of immobility been the initial reason for consultation. To provide merely the obvious means of getting such a person moving might well solve the apparent problems in the short term. Such management could, however, undermine the patient's confidence should it involve unnecessary effort or even the patient's failure. The unidentified barriers to mobility might well be other than those which the patient first presented to the doctor. The professional tasks can be much more rewarding with the detective work. An adequate examination will save time in the long run and prove more satisfying.

WHAT ARE THE COMPONENTS?

Preparation

In order that examination of a patient is effective and economical of time, it is helpful to do a certain amount of information gathering in advance. It does not finish at this point, but is likely to continue as long as the relationship is maintained, since early information can change or new influences arise. Discovering the reason for admission to hospital or consulting the doctor will be the first step, realizing that it is not necessarily the reason for physiotherapy. Often they do coincide, such as in many cases of orthopaedic problems, stroke or some neurological disease. If the reason for referral comes not directly from the patient but a carer, it is usually helpful to establish, as far as possible, the reasons for the referrer's cry for help as it can be unexpected. The nurse, relative or warden of the residential home may, when questioned, report quite specific difficulties of getting out of bed, or falls while walking. Discovery of this may save time that might be involved in a full range of functional testing at first and help to solve the immediate worries early.

3

Example: Mrs Cushion, a resident in a Home, is referred because of 'osteoarthritis'. Medical notes reveal a long account of repeated periods of physiotherapy for most of her arthritic joints. There have been previous strokes and abdominal operations. She has moved only recently from her own house where she had lived alone. It might be assumed that another period of physiotherapy treatment is going to be requested. Discussion with her warden, however, reveals that her own furniture has not yet been delivered, and that the difficulty to the care staff is in helping Mrs Cushion to stand up. Immediately this narrows the field for investigation to the area of sitting and standing for Mrs Cushion herself, the furniture, and handling methods used by care staff. After this she may need no specific treatment for the osteoarthritic joints.

As for a patient of any age, it is necessary to have knowledge of recent and past medical history gleaned from the medical notes or doctor. Previous illnesses or operations may be relevant. Many elderly patients will have accummulated irreversible conditions. Old fractures or strokes or polio may have left residual disability. Mention of recent bereavement or other losses forewarns the physiotherapist to approach such topics carefully. In cases of disturbed communication, whether this be due to deafness, aphasia, dementia or other mental illness, much of the advance information gathering will have to be from notes or a domestic carer.

Current diagnosis and drugs, and information on social background should be noted. Understanding of drugs and compliance is variable. In some cases when the patient is at home it can be useful to discover what is prescribed and to assess how much is taken. Some will have side effects that the physiotherapist should be aware of. As the body ages it becomes less efficient at handling many drugs. Reduced gastric and intestinal motility slows down absorption rates. Some of the liver functions are affected if a drug is not extensively metabolized, the substantial decline in renal function then becomes the major factor in the drugs handling. Multi-pathology which may lead to polypharmacy compounds the difficulty. Important effects that might affect physiotherapy include drowsiness, slowing of reaction time and ataxia (Macdonald, 1985). If there are surprising side effects, the patient needs to be encouraged to discuss them with the prescribing doctor. The physiotherapist should deal with her patient as a whole person with individual background, needs and worries. Advance knowledge of medical and social history from which appropriate details are selected helps provide a starting point

4

that gives the physiotherapist confidence to start the examination appropriately.

The patient's story

It is important to listen to what the patient says as he will provide information not available from other sources. This first contact helps to establish the supportive relationship which could facilitate treatment. Interruptions from any source should be discouraged. Part of the skill of listening to the patient's story lies in paying attention to the ordinary rules of courtesy. If the therapist introduces herself by name, and in the first instance at least, uses the patient's title and surname, any less formal address can be adopted later by agreement. This is more important for some people than others, perhaps particularly for patients whose upbringing or culture has been relatively formal or sheltered. People of an ethnic origin that is unfamiliar to the therapist need particular attention. It may even be necessary to ask how to address that person properly.

On most occasions the reason for referral will be obvious to the patient, but sometimes when the course of the conversation indicates some misunderstanding it may be helpful to ask what he thinks is the reason. In a case of his uncertainty a short introduction to the physiotherapist's area of interest could be helpful in indicating the purpose of the interview.

Unless the patient's main difficulties, or preoccupying symptoms are quite obvious, it is usually helpful to ask him first to indicate where to start the interview. If pain is the chief symptom, then the questioning would follow the conventional pattern to discover its area, intensity, character and behaviour. Even if the patient has an obvious impairment such as a hemiplegia it is still worth finding out what is worrying him at that moment. It might be backache or constipation. To discover what activities are difficult and why, if the patient cannot remember, it might be useful to think through the day's routine or ordinary procedures.

The interviewer should try to keep a logical line of questioning. A rapid change of topic should be avoided lest this lead to confusion. A check list of common items can be used. The physiotherapist should always be aware of using too rigid a format. This can override the therapist/patient relationship and can result in a loss of useful information if it happens not to be on the questionnaire (French, 1988). While the use of too rigid a format can result in loss

5

of useful information, at the same time the therapist can have difficulty in making sense of a variety of information unless there is some habitual sequence of questions. The patient may need guidance in sticking to the main story. One reason is the likely multiplicity of factors that are troublesome, or might limit mobility. Some will be of long standing. Some will be new. If the recall of a day's routine reveals no special information, or is inappropriate, a series of questions could be phrased thus:

'What activity could you manage before . . . that you cannot do now?'
'How long is it since you last . . .?'
'What is it that stops you now?' (There might be several reasons: pain, shortness of breath, stiffness, restriction of the carer, loss of a friend.)

The answer to the last question can be useful to pinpoint. The barriers to independence can be of all kinds, not every one of which will be remediable. This open-ended exploratory interview is the sort of investigation required for patients who have not suffered some obvious disability that needs attention, such as a recent stroke or a single joint problem. At the later stages of rehabilitation or after a gradual decline in mobility, problems are not so easy to identify and certainly not possible without taking the patient's view. His interpretation of the current difficulties leading to his assessment of priorities and expectations on how he will manage should be sought and taken into account when setting goals (see Chapter 3).

Example: Mr Hutson, in trying to explain his difficulty in moving, may reveal by chance or intention that there were problems before admission. He had a fall while walking up the garden only the day before and hurt his back. His present limitation is due to pain quite unconnected with the operation.

Some patients need encouragement to talk. Others, grateful perhaps for the opportunity, pour out a stream of stories. The patient, particularly with the confidence provided by his own home, can have worries, complaints or frustrations that, though they are not of immediate relevance to the present situation, yet have been bottled up awaiting a health service professional who might listen. It seems to be necessary to allow it all to come out, even if nothing can be done about the injury or no explanation be offered for apparent injustices or delays. Only afterwards can the patient concentrate on what the physiotherapist has come for.

6

Separated from the family some patients may give an account of activities that, if not inaccurate, are years out-of-date. Even quite plausible tales of recent independent achievements may need tactful checking with others involved.

Example: Mrs Anderson, in hospital for an infection on top of chronic bronchitis, reports that she walks several miles to do her shopping and does all the housework. It seems unlikely when her flexed hips and shortness of breath make it difficult for her to walk to the toilet, but she might do it, allowing for a little exaggeration of the distance. Then her daughter reveals how frequently she is obliged to help out and the report is revealed to be of years ago.

When the patient is examined at home one or more members of the family may be present. This can be helpful if corroboration of details is required, or if the patient's poor hearing or mental confusion make communication difficult. An embarrassing predicament for the physiotherapist can arise when the family member attempts to conduct a conversation over the patient's head, or makes derogatory statements or accusations about him. Without attempting to answer these, the therapist should acknowledge the feelings expressed with a phrase such as 'I see how you feel'. The concern shown can make the encounter acceptable.

An important part of the patient's story is often his social background and his view of it. Questions may be asked about family and friends, and the frequency of contact. His attitude to them might be inferred from the response made.

If the patient seems slightly agitated, enquiries might be made as to whether he has any anxieties or problems that worry him. There may be some who will be anxious without knowing why, in which case this will influence the manner of treatment in future.

Whether the patient is in his own home or in hospital it is sensible to discover who is the chief carer, if there is one, and make an attempt to meet them. This person's satisfaction with his or her role needs to be ascertained and what other commitments there are, such as young children, a job, or even another elderly dependant. This has to be borne in mind when plans are made.

There is more to communication than just words. Susan Hargreaves has described the effects and emphasized the importance of words matching the behaviour and the value of reading the other's reaction.

Non verbal communication is the key factor in all human behaviour. If there is a disparity between the verbal and non

7

verbal message, the receiver responds to the cues emitted non verbally, but is confused about the real meaning of the message. Usually the positive feelings are expressed verbally while the negative feelings are communicated non verbally. Doubts about the sender's sincerity and credibility are raised and lead to unsatisfactory interaction. (Hargreaves, 1987)

The data of non-verbal behaviour include:

Gesture, facial expression, speed of movement
Voice: tone, breathing
Dress and grooming
Posture and proximity
Listening and the use of silence

A moment's reflection will alert the physiotherapist as to how each of these factors affects communication in every day personal life. Since each has a meaning in context, non-verbal cues of touch and proximity are acceptable between physiotherapist and patient, even while they are not well acquainted but in a physiotherapeutic setting. Positive behaviour includes smiling, a friendly tone of voice and appropriate eye contact. Attention to the patient's comfort which would enable him to concentrate on the interview may be made by adjusting chair or pillows. As this behaviour is observable in both directions, is instant and reliable, encouraging cues have to come from a source of genuine concern or a good actor. Consciousness of the effect of her own behaviour can help a therapist to emphasize her intention to demonstrate good will. Taking note of his, or a family member's behaviour may offer clues about that person's real attitudes. Expressions of intention to be helpful are sometimes belied by the speaker's shifting towards the door rather hastily.

In practical terms, any interview should be conducted at the patient's level, the physiotherapist sitting, if necessary, and within easy contact distance. Care should be taken in making enough eye contact to be reassuring, while not being interpretable as aggressive.

Many professionals are unaware of who cannot see well, but it should be realized that visual impairment renders people less well able to adapt to new faces and places. Even though 1% of people aged 70–79 are registered blind and 5% of those over 85 years, it is thought that a further 30% could be eligible for registration (Cullinan, 1986). For the purposes of a physiotherapist's examination, it is usually necessary only to check that the patient can see his immediate surroundings.

If there are signs of his not taking in what is being said, the need for or positioning of a hearing aid should be checked. It is more important to speak clearly than loudly.

Observation

Much useful information can be gained by conscious observation of a patient and the surroundings. This is increased through interpretive understanding of the effects of disease or disability and experience of individuals.

Even from a distance, observation of a patient's posture may give clues to his state of body or mind; an awkwardly slumped sitting position can arouse suspicion that the patient with a stroke has a disturbance of balance, or perception of body image. On coming closer, the general state of clothing, shoes, personal grooming or hygiene is worth noticing. Remains of food down the front of clothes could indicate he does not see it or does not care, but that might be his customary state. A shirt with buttons fastened to the wrong holes may demonstrate a problem in perception, but a will to try to do the task despite difficulty. Facial expression, skin colour, the state of his hands can give clues to general health, although all unusual signs should be investigated rather than taken at face value. Reactions to the therapist, his concentration and sequence of remarks during the interview should be noted. All observed disabilities may not be important in altering function.

Example: Mrs Howell may have hands grossly deformed by rheumatoid arthritis, but is quite competent to look after herself including the cooking. The same observation on another patient who also has a painful knee will warn the physiotherapist of a possible barrier to the patient's use of walking sticks. In some cases, however, the hands may not look to be greatly affected, but the pain of an inflammatory episode in late-onset rheumatoid arthritis can render the patient almost totally helpless.

Surroundings in an institution will not offer much information on the patient's background, but a photograph or personal possessions can offer clues on family and interests. Observations made in his own home provide more hints. Not only does this make it easier to add a personal touch to the professional relationship, but it might be easier to forecast his expected level of activity by seeing signs of baking in the kitchen, a tended garden or piles of books and newspapers. The state of

9

cleanliness, or supply of food in the larder, may indicate the level of self care.

In hospital, the immediate surroundings will not only be unfamiliar, but possibly inconvenient. In case it turns out to be important, it is worth noting the position of furniture. For a disabled patient access to the bedside locker could be checked in case his reaching it is either painful or impossible. Short distance and convenience of access to the toilet will promote continence – so distance and situation might be crucial.

In any setting the chair in which the patient is seated should be assessed, both for the comfort and support it provides, and as a base from which that patient has the maximal freedom to stand up. The reason for this attention is that many elderly people who become patients are likely both to be sitting for prolonged periods and to have some difficulty in getting up due to an illness, debility or stiffening joints.

The seat of an appropriate chair should provide a firm level base for almost the complete length of the person's thigh. A very soft low-slung seat or one that slopes backward can present an obstacle to his moving forward in preparation for rising. Long periods spent leaning back can upset a patient's posture and balance when he does stand up.

To facilitate the patient's standing up, the height of the chair seat can be of critical importance. In most cases, its height, while bearing the patient's weight, should equal the measurement from the back of his knee to the floor, minus about 1.5 in. (4 cm) to avoid uncomfortable pressure on the back of his thigh. Rising from too low a chair or bed will waste energy, could aggravate knee joint pain and upset confidence, even if the action is possible. The proper use of good arm rests, however, are said to be twice as effective in aiding rising as having a high chair (Ellis, and Munton, 1982). When chair-fast residents of three Social Services Homes were provided with other seating at recommended heights, 77% of them could rise unaided (Finlay et al., 1983).

Depending on the patient's ability, various aspects of the home should be inspected for safety hazards and convenience of access. For anyone with poor eyesight or a difficulty in gait, floor surfaces should be clear of loose items that he might trip over, or if there are fixtures such as a threshold bar, noted in case practice in crossing over should be necessary (see also Chapter 6). An abundance of furniture in a room may be useful for him to lean on as he gets about. If he has to have a walking frame more space might be cleared. The position of the electric or gas switches, could be altered by the appropriate service

10

engineer if he cannot bend down. Access to the garden or road may need to be looked at. Some attention to the level of background noise may be necessary if the patient finds it hard to concentrate or remember. Continuous sound from radio or television while ignored by some, can be very distracting for patients who can cope with only one stimulus at a time.

Finally, it is useful to observe the patient's attitude and reaction to others in the ward, or the personal relationships which exist between patient and carers at home. If there is friction and distress it may need careful enquiry. Sometimes, if this is recent and due to the illness, it can be ameliorated through the effects of treatment and explanations. In any setting there can be a good reciprocal feeling between patient and carer, whether nurse or family member, which can enable both to overcome great difficulties. Long-standing lack of understanding, antipathy or anxiety on the other hand, will probably increase any ill-effect caused by disability or disease. A therapist who notices this will be able to temper her approach accordingly.

Tests

Physiotherapy tests form that part of the examination that helps to measure the patient's level of ability. Ideally all tests should be conducted in a manner that can be repeatable and recorded in terms that can be quantified. Lung function and range of joint motion tests, for example, can be measured by standard methods. The measurement of everyday functional activity is less straightforward due to the difficulty of making the tests realistic for home life in that multiple factors are implicated, and due to quantifying the amount of help that is provided. The conducting of mental tests for perception, memory or depression sometimes needs special aptitudes, including sensitivity and tact. Without tests, however, the presenting level of patient's ability and changes would be hard to demonstrate and impossible to measure. In practice, few physiotherapists undertake extensive tests for perception, though simple ones could be done and results are useful to know. Likewise, mental testing for confusional states or depression should be understood by any therapist, even if conducted by another.

The choice of test, as for a patient of any age, would be according to perceived need. For many an elderly patient the range of tests might be broader, including aspects that he or she would not realize as being affected by an accident or new illness.

11

Figure 1.1 Physical function chart.

Physical Function Chart

Date

1. Bed mobility

2. Transfers - basic
   (Bed - Chair - Commode)

3. Transfers - advanced
   (Toilet - Bath - Car)

4. Balance - sitting 1 minute

5. Balance - standing 1 minute

6. Walking - Depedence indoors

7. Walking aid

8. Walking distance - feet

9. Stairs - number

10. Walking - dependence outdoors

11. Pain level

Key 1-10
1. Independent
2. + Supervision
3. + Minimal guidance
4. + Skilled help
5. Unable

Key 11
1. No pain
2. Present, not limiting
3. Occasionally intereferes with activity
4. Constant/Often interferes
5. Prevents activity

Example: Mr Sewell, having lived for years in an older house, stumbles down a step, which accident causes damage to his back and one shoulder. In addition to checking the areas of pain and the other large joints, it would be as well to check his balance reactions and all the everyday activities that are involved in walking and carrying things. It may often be useful in such a case to do some simple tests of his visual acuity and to assess his level of hearing. It is as well to be aware whether signs such as shortness of breath, or stiff joints are recent or of long standing. In the latter case, measurements should be taken so that the therapist can assess what disabilities the patient is

12

already coping with when she tries to reduce the effects of new impairments.

Tests of everyday functional activity should be appropriate both for that particular patient's ability level and needs which may be discovered by asking questions of him and any involved family member. In practice most patients will need to attempt many of the same daily activities, such as getting out of bed, rising from a chair, standing and walking. For a few there are likely to be special needs: activities that require balance skill, such as hanging out washing or walking over gravel, perhaps across a road. A functional ability chart that records the influence of pain is shown in Figure 1.1. This was adapted in language from a study in the USA on the outcome of physiotherapy with elderly patients (Steffen and Meyer, 1985).

The tests should be started at the level of competence or a little lower for encouragement's sake without going too far in this direction and wasting time. The sequence should be halted before failure seems certain.

If success is in doubt, help should be provided, such as manual assistance in rising from a chair, support in standing to prevent pain, and enough time allowed to give the patient a real chance. If the patient varies in performance from day to day, or morning to evening, and he is planning to return home, tests should be repeated on several occasions. In all cases, an explanation of the purpose of tests should be offered. When the patient is confused, functional tests should be very obviously purposeful. A walk may be to collect a cup of tea, or some other obvious goal. This given reason may need to be repeated during the process to reinforce a failing memory.

For a frail patient, the variety of tests may need to be conducted over a sequence of sessions, the most important being done first. It is questionable whether it is worth moving the patient's position from chair to bed, or even his undressing at the first interview unless signs or history indicate the need to inspect a particular limb. The stress and energy required could reduce his ability to co-operate. Some active and passive movement testing could be conducted in the position in which he is found.

Some patients' response or history giving may indicate some loss of memory or impairment of intellectual function. Assessment of its degree is useful since the outcome of many treatments will be affected by the patient's mental state. It will be underestimated by some observers if the patient's personality is well preserved and conversation seems fluent. It can also be overestimated when inattention or

13

slow reactions are caused by deafness, depression or physical disease (Caird and Judge, 1979).

The conducting of any test of memory or intellectual function should be carefully done, especially if the patient, already aware of some failure, does not wish it to be exposed. In hospital such tests would commonly be carried out by the doctor, but the therapist needs to understand the method and implications of the result.

One validated test that can seem interesting and challenging without being threatening, calls for listing of ten items in four different categories: fruit, towns, colours and animals (Isaacs and Akhtar, 1972). The manner of completion, whether reflective or hasty, repetitively or in other confused fashion can also be informative. The test requires alertness, concentration and short-term memory, but is not heavily dependent on the subject's cultural background. A maximum score would be ten for each set.

When a patient persistently fails to respond due to apparent apathy, it is not always easy to differentiate depression from some forms of dementia, including that associated with Parkinsonism. A few simple queries about interests, attitude to life and whether sleeping habits have changed, may point to abnormal low spirits. Members of the family may have noticed changes. Other members of staff should also be consulted for their observations on his behaviour. 'Normal' levels of unhappiness for known reasons should not, of course, be confused with clinical depression. There are simple screening tests available which help determine whether the patient should be investigated fully by a specialist doctor. One questionnaire designed specifically for use with the older patient has been described by Yesavage and Brink (1983) (Figure 1.2). It does not require a trained interviewer, but certainly one who would offer total attention and sympathy. Depression in elderly people is not always recognized, especially by the general practitioner (Williamson, 1981) who perhaps does not see the patient for long enough at any one visit.

At the end of any examination, however brief or extensive, the patient should be offered the physiotherapy diagnosis, and as much explanation as he wishes. Table 1.1 gives a check list of possible tests.

Assessment

Assessment is an intellectual exercise on the part of the physiotherapist; an interpretation of the findings during examination in order to make a decision on what should happen next. Often the

14

Figure 1.2 Geriatric depression scale.

GERIATRIC DEPRESSION SCALE

PATIENT'S NAME: .... D.O.B.: ....

DATE: .... WARD: .... DIAGNOSIS: ....

Choose the best answer for how you felt over the past week.

1. Are you basically satisfied with your life? .... YES/*NO
2. Have you dropped many of your activities and interests? .... *YES/NO
3. Do you feel that your life is empty? .... *YES/NO
4. Do you often get bored? .... *YES/NO
5. Are you hopeful about the future? .... YES/*NO
6. Are you bothered by thoughts you cannot get out of your
   head .... *YES/NO
7. Are you in good spirits most of the time? .... YES/*NO
8. Are you afraid something bad is going to happen to you? ..... *YES/NO
9. Do you feel happy most of the time? .... YES/*NO
10. Do you often feel helpless? .... *YES/NO
11. Do you often get restless and fidgety? .... *YES/NO
12. Do you prefer to stay at home, rather than going out and
    doing new things? .... *YES/NO
13. Do you frequently worry about the future? .... *YES/NO
14. Do you feel you have more problems with memory than
    most? .... *YES/NO
15. Do you think it is wonderful to be alive now? .... YES/*NO
16. Do you often feel downhearted and blue? .... *YES/NO
17. Do you feel pretty worthless the way you are now? .... *YES/NO
18. Do you worry a lot about the past? .... *YES/NO
19. Do you find life very exciting? .... YES/*NO
20. Is it hard for you to get started on new projects? .... *YES/NO
21. Do you feel full of energy? .... YES/*NO
22. Do you feel that your situation is hopeless? .... *YES/NO
23. Do you think that most people are better off than you are? ... *YES/NO
24. Do you frequently get upset over little things? .... *YES/NO
25. Do you frequently feel like crying? .... *YES/NO
26. Do you have trouble concentrating? .... *YES/NO
27. Do you enjoy getting up in the morning? .... YES/*NO
28. Do you prefer to avoid social gatherings? .... *YES/NO
29. Is it easy for you to make decisions? .... YES/*NO
30. Is your mind as clear as it used to be? .... YES/*NO

Rating Scales		Mark 1 point for those asterisked
normal	0-9	TOTAL: ....
mild depressive	10-19	
severe depressive	20-30	THERAPIST: ....

PATIENT'S COMMENTS: THERAPIST'S COMMENTS:

Table 1.1 Check list of possible tests

Communication
Complete tests in this section would commonly be undertaken by others, but a simple exploratory trial done by a physiotherapist can reveal whether or not this patient should be referred on.
Speech: receptive ability, expressive ability
Hearing: acuity
Visual: acuity, field
Mental: intellectual function, depression.

Cardiovascular and respiratory systems

Respiratory rate	Peak expiratory flow rate
Pulse	Forced expiratory volume
Chest expansion	Exercise tolerance
Auscultation	

Locomotor system
Joint range of movement: active, passive range
physiological, accessory
Joint alignment
Muscle length
Muscle strength
Limb length
Limb girth

Nervous system
Pain appreciation: subjective examination, observation of behaviour
Skin sensation: touch, pressure, temperature
Joint sense: position, direction of movement
Perception: awareness and interpretation of body, space, habitual activity, sensation, relationships of objects (many occupational therapists are skilled at this, but physiotherapists should know the common tests).
Tendon reflexes
Quality of movement control
Muscle tone
Balance reactions: righting and equilibrium

Functional activity
As appropriate - see also Figure 1.1
Urinary continence

purpose is to analyse the collected information in order to select the patient's real problems, to identify which ones might be helped by physiotherapy, and to make a plan of management and treatment. Sometimes a professional opinion is requested by a doctor, or perhaps a warden of a residential home, on whether physiotherapy has anything at all to offer in a particular case. Assessment is based on the results of the examination and assisted by clear record keeping. Experience of other patients and discussion with colleagues are likely to help in the analysis. Although it is common practice to focus on the problems a patient may present, it is worthwhile registering his assets also, whether personal or environmental. The assessment of a patient's being able to live safely or comfortably at home will take into consideration the condition of the house, availability or fitness of a principal carer, and probably the patient's own mental competence and determination.

Example: Mrs Ames has for years had a great struggle to get about her old house because of arthritic joints and obesity. A small stroke with some loss of joint sensation causes her to be unsafe going to the toilet or getting in and out of bed.

It may seem at first assessment as if she would have to consider moving to a residential home. Only when the advantages of a numerous and helpful young family next door, who arrange to supervise dangerous activities, and her own optimism are taken into account does the whole assessment alter.

Affluent patients and those with fond relations who live nearby are more frequently enabled to be at home helped by paid assistants and the convenience of comfortable accommodation. However, even people well educated in every other aspect of life often still need the support and advice that physiotherapists can provide.

A physiotherapist should be aware of the risk of making false assumptions about a patient's needs or style of living, especially should it be different from her own. Standards desired by the patient are likely to be based on the level he is accustomed to. What may seem like intolerable shabbiness, inconvenience or gloom to a visitor may not be deemed a disadvantage in the patient's estimation. What may be more important in environmental terms would be access to warmth, appropriate furniture and the kindliness of neighbours, or a regular visitor.

A difficult point in assessment for physiotherapy can be in the balance of priority in the patient's needs. When the patient is in hospital this might be whether he has the capacity to recover if a full rehabilitation programme is undertaken, or whether for reasons of frailty or pathology he would be more suited to a scheme to maintain him in comfort at his maximum current functioning. Another balance of priority of needs might be which of his signs and symptoms are most important – whether they are life threatening, whether likely to lead to a fixed deformity or increased discomfort, or whether

17

reversible. At home, the balance might be between the needs of a would-be active patient who nevertheless requires supervision and those of a wife with other demands on her time, or her own disability to cope with. In considering these it will be helpful to listen to the various points of view from other therapists, the family and the relevant doctor.

Once an assessment of problems, assets and various needs is made in collaboration with others, the programme of care can be more easily decided. The initial assessment may change in the light of events, but is a reference point and basis for physiotherapy contribution to the multidisciplinary team decision.

Decision making

The decisions to be made are about the general aim of management to be proposed to the rest of the team and what specific goals might be discussed with the patient and others. Then follows a choice of physiotherapy measures that might be considered and the urgency, timing and manner in which they should be carried out. In some cases thought will be given about referral of the patient to other agencies (social services, voluntary organization) or to professional people (therapists). Plans may be made for liaison with people outside hospital (home help, district nurse).

In the case of a patient for whom active measures are to be chosen, the selection of these will relate to the findings of the examination and tests. The manner of approach may need consideration if the patient is perhaps confused or very deaf and the style should be sensitive to the response obtained. If the judgement has been made that active rehabilitation is inappropriate for a particular patient, decisions may have to be made on particular needs. Some attention might be required to promote his comfort or to plan secondary prevention of problems that might be caused by prolonged recumbency. In collaboration with ward staff or the occupational therapist, the best choice of furniture or fixed supports in the toilet are part of treatment in general terms. Tests will have revealed what activities can be encouraged, what requires personal help or that a walking aid should be selected. Experience of long-term disability as well as knowledge of pathological conditions will enable decisions to be taken on the sort of difficulties that might require preventive measures. Frequency of inspection in future will need to be determined to check and prevent such possibilities as joint or soft tissue contracture, or unnecessary loss of function.

Sometimes a decision will be made that physiotherapy would have nothing to offer in which case this is explained both to the patient and the referrer.

Recording

The act of writing down a physiotherapist's findings and opinions is one that many find extremely tedious or difficult. Nevertheless, it is absolutely essential for a number of reasons, does not have to be extensive and should, in fact, be selective and as brief as is consistent with its purpose. The process of recording can also help in the thought processes of assessment and planning (see p. 130). The purposes of record keeping are for evaluation, to ensure legality, and the passing of information to others.

Evaluation

Memory itself is neither adequate nor valid in assessing or reporting patients' progress. Whether for monitoring change over time as a basis for treatment decisions or for the purposes of research, accurate records must be kept at the time of care.

Legality

In cases of litigation a reasoned account of treatment should be available, and one that could be read and understood by another physiotherapist.

Transmission of information

The progress of patients who are in long-term care, or who are shifted from one institution to another, or to the supervision of community physiotherapists should be accompanied by records that provide appropriate advice. Continuing physiotherapy management will be assisted by notes on the current aims, measures and achievements, with dates.

The Problem Oriented Medical Record is one system that is being adapted for physiotherapy purposes and is becoming widely used. The whole system includes the record, audits and the education programme which is based on the first two items.

19

The recording system consists of:

Data base
Problem list
Plans
Progress notes
Discharge summary

The *data base* includes the personal information and medical history, the patient's account and physiotherapy findings. For clarity, the clinical details are grouped under the following sections:

'S' The subjective data include comments of the patient or other interested party.

'O' The objective data consist of the medical history the physiotherapist's measurements and observations. Some of this is most clearly set out in charts.

'A' The assessment is the professional opinion which may be a diagnosis of the origin of pain, the chief assets or barriers to recovery, perhaps a prognosis. The use of asterisks in the 'S' and 'O' sections can help to draw attention to salient points.

'P' The plan of treatment usually consists of physiotherapy measures, e.g. electrical treatment dosages, activities, and contacts to be made.

The *problem list* is simply a list of the patient's difficulties, physical, mental, social and practical, in order to keep them in perspective. They are listed as active or inactive and referred to by number elsewhere in the notes as they are addressed (Table 1.2).

The plans are drawn up to meet (a) the overall aim of management and (b) goals and objectives to be achieved (Chapter 3).

The *progress notes* need only be quite brief, recording merely changes. Whenever appropriate the quickest means is to use a chart which can be marked. Any new information should be marked as relevant by initials S.O.A.P in the margin, and by the problem number (Table 1.3).

The *discharge summary* is particularly useful when a patient is transferred to another physiotherapist's care in drawing to her attention the up-to-date thinking on aims of physiotherapy in this case. When a patient is re-admitted, the previous summary can be a useful basis for reconsidering plans, assuming the overall problem list is much the same. If the patient is discharged to a residential home, precise information should be sent about his activity level and particular needs such as furniture heights or toilet aids. Figure 1.3

20

Table 1.2 Problem list

Date	No.	Active	Inactive	Physiotherapist's initials
3.3.88	1	OA lumbar spine back pain		
	2		Rt. below knee amputation 1986	
	3	Unable to transfer alone		
6.3.88	4	Acute chest infection on chronic bronchitis	15.3.88	
16.3.88	5	Daughter out all day		£ℳ𝓈

Table 1.3 Progress notes

Date	No.		
4.3.88	1	S	Backache ↓ while sitting, lying ↑ after standing 30 seconds
		O	Chair ↙ Seems drowsy. Function - see chart
		A	Unwell - not unwilling
		P	Apply Rt. prosthesis. Assist standing briefly
7.3.88	4	O	SOB difficulty in expectoration
		P	Alt. side ly., breathing exercises + shaking if necessary.
16.3.88	1, 3	S	Backache ↓ standing 2 minutes
		O	Function - see chart
		P	Contact daughter re discharge needs. Encourage stand, walk + support.

gives a suggested front page of notes which includes space for a discharge summary.

A more complete guide to record keeping is provided by the Documentation and Retrieval Group of the Chartered Society of Physiotherapy (1988) (*see* pp. 111–14).

Review

Patients with physical disability are often kept under long-term surveillance by a physiotherapist. For those permanently in long-term care in an institution, or at home, even those in a slow-stream rehabilitation programme, a review of current activity should be reconsidered at intervals. Short-term review is also used for those patients recently discharged from hospital, but who are considered vulnerable to change, e.g. patients with Parkinson's disease or other

21

Figure 1.3 Suggested front page of notes including space for a discharge summary.

NHS No.		FIP No.		ADDRESS	
Surname					
Forename				Tel.	
Occupation		DOB		G.P.	
Unit		Location			
Consultant		Speciality		Tel.	
Diagnosis		Code		G.P. Code	
Ref. by		Reason		Code	Appliance
D/C		End Status		Trans-action	Outcome
Transport: Str. Ch. Wk. Man.				Audit	
Assessment Date				Physiotherapist	
Support Services	S.W. D.N.				
	R.O. H.H. M.O.W.				
Social Situation					
In patient Out patient	Mobility W/C Aids Home visit YES/NO Report YES/NO				
Discharge summary					
				Total number Treatments	

Source: Physiotherapy Service, Greenwich Health District (unpublished).

balance problems who might lose confidence. Reviews should be conducted with reference to goal planning (Chapter 3).

In long-term surveillance it cannot be assumed that absolute levels of health and activity can be unvarying since, apart from the natural deterioration due to disease or forced immobility which takes its toll, there could be new illnesses, accidents or other affecting events. In practice only those people just coping as on a knife edge of independence tend to be checked. Some patients can be supplied with the name and telephone number of a therapist and encouraged to call if need arises.

Even if the patient has no new apparent injury, other events can alter his situation and ability; staff in an institution will change, he moves to another room or building, a close friend or a member of the family dies. Any of these can have an impact for good or ill. The less physically or mentally independent a patient is the more he is vulnerable to external changes.

Outpatient or domiciliary review is often arranged soon after any period of intensive treatment to foster confidence and pick up on any unexpected difficulties or misunderstandings. Frequently it will depend on a number of factors; distance from the physiotherapy base, perceived need and prognosis. If there is another therapist, district nurse or health visitor involved, liaison might be maintained.

The first part of any review would be taken up with discovering any fresh developments in patient's life, and his impression of how he is coping. This would need corroboration by other parties if there is any indication that he might be unrealistic in his judgement.

To be economical of time, and to make a valid comparison, it would be sensible to test the same activities under the previous conditions at each review. For the purposes of encouragement, any home exercises need to be checked, including the practical details of frequency, safety, and convenience of home conditions for their practice (see pp. 152-3).

For patients in continuing care wards or at home, quite often a management regime has to be considered in the light of new conditions. New staff may need advice on handling, and lower activity levels may be agreed. There is no need for despondency in a case such as this. It is probably kindest to the patient to change plans on the evidence of a thorough review, not necessarily to maintain the most strenuous programme, but to adapt to a more realistic one. On some occasions increased confidence or another factor will have led to improvement.

23

HOW IS IT DIFFERENT WITH OLDER PATIENTS?

An examination should be conducted on any patient, irrespective of age, before an assessment of needs can properly be made. The choice of how and where to collect information and the selection of tests will be related to the condition of the patient. Adaptation of behaviour in dealing with an adult is influenced by the patient's personality, his mental powers and the capacity of the examiner.

Reasons

The physiotherapist should be aware of the need to modify her examination with respect to the old-age-related aspects of patients. These include the possibility of multiple pathology, the social effect of age and experience difference between the physiotherapist and patient, and the natural physiological changes of ageing. In some patients these aspects may seem apparently negligible, and in others quite daunting, but it helps to remember that the person behind the exterior has very similar personal needs as one of any age, including acknowledgement of his individuality.

It is possible for those who work in hospitals to forget that there are plenty of elderly people who cope independently and socially almost to the end of their days. Nevertheless, if such a healthy individual arrived in a physiotherapy department with a minor injury, there will be some added features that a careful physiotherapist will take into account during examination.

Effects

Examination and assessment of older patients needs to be more extensive and conducted more slowly and sensitively with an informed awareness of social background and history.

The extent of the investigation may include a wider physical and mental examination than the initially presenting reason would indicate. Details of physical environment and social network may be helpful to know in both the current period and recent past. Sometimes there are questions about more distant past injuries and illness to be asked.

A child or young person with known multiple disability would require extensive examination, but the primary signs and symptoms

24

are likely to have arisen from a single if complicated source such as cerebral palsy, a severe neurological illness or accident. The needs in an older person may not be immediately obvious because some of them will be apparently of minor importance and unconnected. The relevance is to do with the insidious effect on a patient's active life, and for the physiotherapist the value of gaining the most complete story.

Mrs Jewson, (section 'Why examine') might offer her knees to be looked at. In addition to the conventional examination of knee joints in both their passive and active state and how this affects daily life, enquiries can be made on the condition during recent months before seeing the physiotherapist. She may have been out and about and undertaking household tasks or alternatively living in a much less physically active way for years. Limitations to activity other than painful knees such as a lung or heart condition or recent significant alteration to mental state or social situation may need checking.

The incidence of multiple mobility difficulties for the elderly has been well documented. In a survey of 1600 older people at home, those aged 65–74 years suffered an average of 4.6 chronic conditions (Abrams, 1978). Half of these number suffered from arthritis/rheumatism. The other conditions reported by about a third of the sample included poor eyesight, giddiness and breathlessness. For those aged 75 and over the average number of conditions was 5.8. However, 10% reported no physical problems.

In Williamson's (1981) survey, 70% of the sample were discovered to have unreported foot problems. No physiotherapist examining an elderly patient should be surprised at discovering a physical or mental condition unreported to or found by the doctor. It has been suggested that patients tend to report to the doctor only those problems they hope can be ameliorated or in which the latter has indicated an interest (Williamson et al., 1987). Nor should she fail to check all relevant aspects of mobility, whether or not her attention has been drawn to them. For example, a quick check of weight-bearing joints, including shoulders, in someone presenting with a stroke is always sensible. Awareness of a painful joint will affect decisions about treatment. Some signs may be noticed that have been present, but untroubling for many years, such as deformities of posture, a fixed joint, or old polio, but only late in life do they begin to be significantly disabling.

Apart from present clinical problems and accumulated pathology, examination in some cases may need to include other background. In the case of a young disabled person this will include his living

25

environment and perhaps education or work opportunities. The additional factors affecting ease of mobility for an older person relate to the state of housing. Elderly people living on small incomes may become accustomed to shabbier and colder buildings than many a physiotherapist would tolerate. Issues of safety are discussed in Chapter 6.

The importance of social support is in proportion to the patient's level of dependence. Coping with life despite illness, disability or general frailty may be achieved with help from others. Identification of the type of help to assist activity falls not only to the physiotherapist, but her awareness of other factors of independence is necessary, such as the encouragement that can only be provided by people.

All through life most people live as part of a social network, as contributors and beneficiaries. When a child, others are older and more capable. In middle years, there will be maximal social opportunity and few will have none to turn to for help. Very elderly people quite often have fewer friends, and these may be equally old and frail. There may be no immediate or local family or the spouse may be equally feeble. The gaps may need to be filled by one younger relation, neighbours or a worker for the social services. Some older people are unaware of their dependency, but physiotherapists should not be surprised at the level of anxiety about the burden of responsibility (fears of falls being one) felt by some carers, and may have to be prepared to listen to their worries also. Some of these will tell a quite different tale to the patient about how much he accomplishes. The long duration of some relationships and the resulting level of attachment may be important. Old friends or old spouses may either have grown closer or even more disenchanted with each other. In the first case affection can overcome enormous obstacles; in the second, added disability can be the last straw that causes the carer to give up. This must be taken into the overall assessment as to whether an in-patient may be discharged, or when he seems not to be making expected progress at the day hospital.

The slow speed of conducting an examination may be necessary for a variety of reasons with older patients. Very few people take in or remember all that is said in a hospital setting, due to differences in education background, the strange setting, apprehension and nervousness (Wagstaff, 1982). Comprehension may be slower in advanced age. Some of this effect will be due to the reasons just mentioned. Added factors which relate to some elderly patients are lowered hearing acuity, especially for high tones, some

26

slowing both in central processing and peripheral nerve conduction time. There is said to be a 20% increase in reaction time between adults of around 20 and 60 years affecting movements and memory recall (Birren and Woods, 1985). So explanation and questions should allow for reaction time. The time necessary for undressing or moving about may also be longer.

The need for extra sensitivity required by the physiotherapist is to do with stresses felt by most older people, whether or not in hospital. Repeated bereavements take a physical as well as mental toll. There can be losses of places and activities as well as people. There are many other reasons for feeling stress in old age whether or not this is recognized by the older person. Those related to the physiotherapist's examination include the possible long duration of illness, the low status offered by society in general, and the possibility of being on a ward labelled 'geriatric', a name not always understood or appreciated. Older people are said to have a reduced capacity for adapting to changes, though this would vary with individual personalities and experiences (Wattis and Church, 1986). Social customs have changed in the use of titles and surnames, and not all patients feel comfortable with the use of first names, especially without their permission. This could be particularly important for Asian patients. The usual social status of a person in an institution is not at first obvious, but someone who has been used to a professional's life or lived in seclusion or comfort can gain a reputation for being demanding which can be a result of misunderstanding. He may always have been a difficult character, of course, but a change of situation late in life is not easy to adapt to.

27

2

The patient as a person

A key point in good practice by a physiotherapist requires recognition of the patients' needs to regain or maintain personal autonomy and to aim for increasing personal responsibility for recovery.

WHAT IS PERSONAL AUTONOMY?

Standards of professional behaviour assume that chartered physiotherapists will respect the rights, dignity and individual sensibilities of all their patients. This includes a recognition of the need to consider the factors that allow or promote personal autonomy, including the opportunity to consent or decline treatment (Chartered Society of Physiotherapy, 1986).

Personal autonomy implies the power to choose, or to stretch out deliberately towards something within our power. This definition has been elaborated by Dr Mary Warnock with reference to elderly people and the significance of power (Warnock, 1983). Making a choice is dependent on having power to act or react before one can make a choice to stretch out accordingly.

Choosing to walk about or undertake physical activity can be limited by failing health or strength. A person of 90 years of age would not be able to walk as far as someone of 20, both being healthy and normally fit. The possession of money which implies power, provides more options for choice. If the 90 year old can pay for transport he might journey any distance the youngster could manage on foot. People who are elderly, disabled and poor are limited in their scope of activity.

Nearly every person even without money can make choices in how to behave, although he may not exercise it. At his most restricted

28

scope of choice a disabled person can decide how to act, or how to react to others. Some individuals use this power to their own advantage despite being physically inactive, although this does depend on the features of the relationship. Less influential people may try to affect others, but any attempt to achieve some personal autonomy can be suppressed or ignored by more powerful people. Some physiotherapists may not realize quite how much influence they wield in this respect and should try to be sensitive to the efforts of unassertive patients.

Behaviour to some extent seems to be in response to the perceived social norms. We act generally as others expect of us, not only in social customs and courtesies, but in the fulfilling of a role, whether that be post-office clerk, schoolmaster or hospital patient. It is possible to avoid acting in one's usual character; for an adult to perform bizarre or childish actions, for an apparently timid person to act boldly in response to bullying, though either might have to endure the surprise reactions of others. Without confidence it is not always easy to persuade another of one's individuality, especially for timid people away from home surroundings. A patient in hospital tends to adopt the role of passive receiver of treatment and orders, in some cases beyond necessity. From the hospital staff point of view it can be hard to discern usual character and real wishes due to misunderstanding caused by a patient's apparent passivity or stubborn resistance.

Some patients quite undeservedly are seen as anxious, hostile or introverted through a lack of facial expression. As gesture and facial movements are largely interpreted subconsciously, their reduction may give false impressions of mood or intellect and cause the observer to make erroneous judgement of personality. This was shown in a trial when 90 therapists recorded their first impressions of patients with either Parkinson's disease or ischaemic heart disease. Responses to the former group labelled them all as less participative and overall less likeable, although usual psychological testing showed no reason for this. The writers suggested that all health professionals need to take account of their first impressions of Parkinsonian patients, consider the role non-verbal signals have had in their formation and guard against over hasty assumptions about mood, personality and intellect (Pentland et al., 1987).

29

Ageist beliefs

These are really a form of prejudice which can be applied unthinkingly to those of any age: 'too young to be responsible', 'too middle-aged to indulge in such games'. Some people manage both to ignore comments and prove them wrong. Ageist beliefs cause the limiting expectations that are imposed on and adopted by elderly people, which include ill health, disinclination to be active and a reduction of outside interests and hobbies. The outcome is the 'What can you expect at my age' syndrome. There may be some truth in any stereotype, but if adopted totally by an elderly person it is likely to be self-fulfilling. Friends, family and especially health workers if zealously over-caring and pessimistic in outlook could foster unnecessary levels of dependency and the perpetuation of these beliefs.

The easiest time to achieve this is when a person's morale or strength is diminished by accident or period of ill health, by loss of partner, friend or home. At this period sympathy and practical help are usually gladly offered and thankfully received. Many recover from the blow, gradually re-adjust if necessary to new circumstances and re-assert themselves to pick up whichever threads of life are available, maybe even find new ones. Ageist beliefs on the part of younger family or friends, as well as the recipient of help can limit the scope of autonomy if an inappropriate level of help is not withdrawn or the choice to be even a little independent is not allowed.

The role of the physiotherapist lies in explaining the cause of residual disability to patient and family and offering realistic guidance on how much activity to expect or encourage.

Cultural factors

Some cultural factors that affect maintenance of personal autonomy are to do with other belief systems and accustomed life styles. In many families from other parts of Europe, the West Indies and East Africa and Asia who perpetuate the traditional attitudes to their older members, personal autonomy in relation to physical independence may not be required. It may be fostered in other ways such as in the provision of a role with high status and by deference to his opinion and wishes. This should be taken note of by the physiotherapist in planning treatment goals. It may not be necessary for a returning elder to be independent in self care, but more important that his dignity be preserved.

30

People who have had social advantages of an autonomous professional or personal life style may insist on the perpetuation of such independence, and in hospital such determination can cause friction unless the background is appreciated. Those who have always been at the receiving end of employer or landlord, parent or spouse relations, may have lower expectations of autonomy and rehabilitation prospects.

Finance

To some extent, independence will have been affected by financial wealth and stability. The current state of the individual's finances affects opportunities in housing, domiciliary support and transport. Adequate wealth will enable adaptations to be made or change of dwelling undertaken on the patient's own terms. Employment of staff may allow continued life at home where this would otherwise not be possible. There are always some people who have unrealistic expectations of how much money can buy in terms of health. This affects physiotherapy in so far as the therapist takes these into account in assessing the patient's personality for planning treatment goals and deciding when they have been accomplished as well as possible.

Institutionalization

This is the term used to describe the manner of organization within any community which lives or works together, the former situation being most powerful in its effects on the people involved because no other sort of life is being experienced. When the system is managed for the convenience and efficiency of the organization rather than the original purpose of education or health care, then the people for whom it is managed become of secondary importance. This can result in block treatment and fixed routines with little or no allowance being made for individuals. This can lead to social distancing between staff and residents which has a depersonalizing effect on both groups.

Thus the regime in an institution, whether residential home or hospital, is a powerful force for diminishing or promoting personal autonomy of the residents. One sign of a regime that discourages these people is a tidy room but no activity or conversation. Another is the failure of staff to take enough notice of those receiving help.

31

If during an episode of care such as an assisted walk or bath, when that person might hope for some personal attention, the staff talk only to each other over his head, the effect on the patient can only be demoralizing. If without thought, sympathy or recent knowledge, different staff members voice quite fixed and perhaps unrealistic expectations of the residents' ability – 'No-one is allowed rest on their beds/Everyone has to walk to the dining area' – some of the latter may cease to make so much effort to be active.

Similarly, if all staff members have different methods of the physical handling of a resident, confusion and diminished co-operation must result unless, of course, he speaks up for himself and that can cause difficulties. Without individual attention the will on the part of the disabled resident to be independent and to exercise choice will be diminished.

Roger Clough has described, on the basis of extended observation, the difficulties of living in such a public place as a residential home for elderly people, including the influences that limit autonomy (Clough, 1981). He emphasized the importance of the initial impressions received by the manner of welcome and information given, which affected lasting attitudes in several residents. Ideas received about the liberty to use the bedroom as a sitting place, or how much liberty to walk about were retained. Rules were sometimes assumed to exist, but not questioned, so that residents felt unable to break what they perceived as the social norms. It was suggested that in homes where residents' opinions were sought on matters that concerned them in daily life, the atmosphere would be more lively, and initiative would result in greater activity.

The importance of this factor in physiotherapy, apart from ethical considerations, is in the gaining of maximum benefit from the treatment. In encouraging maximal autonomy in rehabilitation or maintenance of physical activity, there will be a good chance of gaining co-operation, raised morale, and a realistic agreement of goals. The patient can feel able to voice ideas on how he might cope, and to take more initiative in practising exercises. From the physiotherapist's point of view, there could be a greater interest in developing areas of choice for the patient, and satisfaction in fostering his confidence. All this is based on the assumption that age has no influence on most peoples' wish to be independent and contributing members of society.

The effect of suppressing autonomy is an over-submissive patient who gives no trouble, but becomes inactive and perhaps morose. This mood affects others at the time, but later the inactivity is likely to give trouble to the staff as he becomes physically dependent. This is more likely if the patient has communication difficulties due to aphasia, dementia, blindness or deafness.

There are limits to the extent of personal autonomy for anyone, however. These are set in society by others' needs and claims. The right of other residents in the institution may need protection when one person is unduly assertive or intrusive. At home, the way of life or feelings of other family members have to be considered by health care professionals who are advocates for the patient. Those patients whose behaviour is self-destructive or foolish may need restraint, but it can be difficult to know quite when and how much to pursue this line without discussion including all interested parties. Individuals have a right to self determination unless a doctor decides that the balance of mind is disturbed, and he is a potential source of danger to others.

Physical and mental disability

These factors need not reduce a person's power to make some choices, although it may affect the power to achieve all desires. He may be obliged to look for help in achieving some wishes and therefore cannot be independent. Serious ill health reduces the options for autonomy considerably, but even then special equipment may be available to enable the person to change the environment such as switching lights on and off.

Environmental barriers

Autonomy can be limited by environmental barriers if, for example, steps are numerous or too steep to be climbed or doors are kept locked. Public awareness of the limited access to buildings, transport and on roads for those in wheelchairs, is being increased slowly through the efforts of those who are restricted. Cot sides on hospital beds are very seldom used now, but a very low chair is a restriction. Those who are confused are usually best restrained from dangerous wandering by distraction or persuasion.

HOW MAY AUTONOMY BE ENCOURAGED BY A PHYSIOTHERAPIST?

There are always people of independent spirit who need no encouragement to make decisions for themselves. One of the main ways of fostering personal autonomy when it is necessary is by means of listening to each person because he is regarded as a valuable human being whose needs will be respected. The areas where this is important in physiotherapy are in the discovery of the patient's assets, in developing his potential and in helping the members of the caring team both family and professionals by sharing knowledge and teaching of handling skills.

Individual attention

Whenever possible patients should be given the opportunity to be in control of their own movements and behaviour. When someone is in the unfamiliar territory of a hospital or is encountering unusual bodily sensation due to illness, information has to be provided to enable decisions to be taken. People need to know the lay-out of the ward or department for example, in order to find their way to a particular room. They need to know the system of appointments, to know the names of relevant people and whom to ask. Most patients need to have their clinical condition explained, perhaps repeatedly. If they are to make decisions on treatment, the options have to be explained with the possible benefits or adverse side effects, and the time scale of the course of treatment estimated.

There are few opportunities for choice where some in-patients are concerned, but a physiotherapist should be able to assess where this is possible. For one patient this might be the time of treatment, for another in which direction to walk or perhaps to select an alternative of two activities.

A patient who has been physically disabled and dependent on help for a long time should always be consulted on how he likes to be handled. Aggressive reaction to what seems to the patient like too much regimentation or bossiness can often be deflected by explanation of options for choice or even just listening to his grumbles. Just allowing him to choose to see the physiotherapist later, or even to let off steam without being ignored, will clear the way for useful intervention. A patient may still refuse treatment despite all attempts at explanation and persuasion. It may be worth finding out from another knowledgeable person if there is a known but perhaps temporary reason for this, such as recent bad news. The physiotherapist may after discussion agree with the patient that it does not seem necessary or worth the effort. In some cases the patient will change his mind at a later date. The therapist must also consider, while attempting to motivate the patient, whether the goal is realistically obtainable with effort, and whether the therapeutic end justifies the means to achieve it. When, if ever, is it permissible to lie to a patient – to say without good reason that he will recover ability? Such ethical considerations, including the problem of the inveterately non-compliant patient, have been outlined by Julius Sims. He questions whether their refusal to co-operate abrogates the right to treatment (Sims, 1983). In practice each case would be considered on the basis of an individual set of facts. Physiotherapy can rarely be carried out if the patient is unwilling and then only passive chest treatment, and when he is in no fit state to make the choice. If the patient is persistantly unwilling, so long as this is discussed with the doctor who has overall clinical responsibility for the case there is not necessarily any need to continue.

In applying the principles of informed consent to patient care, 'The patient's moral right to self determination and the corresponding duty of health professions to do no harm, create a strong moral basis for gaining a patient's informed consent' (Purtillo, 1984). The 'informed consent' depends on the adequacy of information provided and whether the person is capable of deciding rationally about the decision at hand. The next of kin is usually considered the most qualified to make such a judgement on behalf of an incompetent patient and even then the decision should be made with extreme caution.

Occasionally there will be a patient who refuses help because he says he wants to die. However this is voiced, whether quietly, publicly or lightly, this should not be brushed aside jokingly, with dismissive reproof or silence. The patient may or may not wish to enlarge on the topic, explain the reasons or make a cry for help in daily life. If he is generous, serious or courageous enough to tell, the listener will not have to offer any advice or comment. Just to hear someone through when he needs it is an assertion of his importance. This is not an easy task. It is extremely hard to sit and listen to someone without interrupting. Physiotherapists are used to spending a large proportion of their time talking to patients, so learning to listen can be especially difficult. When listening intelligently there are points for attention such as repeated phrases, emotive words or what is not being said. Sometimes they can be followed up. Counselling is essentially a listening process to help patients identify problems and possibly to offer support, but it needs learning and practice (Lawler, 1988).

Sometimes it may be appropriate to ask if there is any particular thing he fears or finds uncomfortable. There may be symptoms of pain or sickness he dreads or even an unknown prognosis in which case a special interview with the doctor might be suggested. Occasionally a firm or concrete wish to achieve an action will be elicited. It may be possible to do something or even just talk about it. If appropriate and desired by the patient, this listening service could be referred to a priest or social worker. This kind of respect for feelings may do much to restore another's faith in the best of human nature, though it came only from one person.

Two-way communication is achieved in all human converse when the manner is appropriate and both are willing. It is, of course, quite different within each family, between strangers, and any mixture one could think of. In order to assist the other to respond sensibly the physiotherapist has to be aware of special difficulties that might be present when conversing with any patient and react appropriately. If it is likely that the other has poor hearing or vision, approach should be made from the front and with warning by touch or expression that something is about to happen. Having checked that she can be seen, the therapist should at all times speak clearly. With a patient who has poor short-term memory, language would have to be in simple phrases, spoken more slowly than usual and perhaps repeated to reinforce its impact and encourage a voluntary response.

All patients should be treated as if rational if for no other reason than it is likely they understand a good deal more than might be expected from their responses. When communication is difficult it is easier to understand the patient's character from responses if some background information has already been gained. Knowledge of clinical data, interests and usual behaviour helps the therapist to see him in the round. Most often this is gained by customary examination and during the development of the therapeutic relationship, no matter how brief. From her side, the therapist must offer acceptance and empathy without being judgemental however surprising any patient's expressed views may be. If thought to be useful, reasons for these views might be invited and these could help to explain behaviour and guide the physiotherapist in planning management.

For some, information on personality through his reactions to other people may be gained if he is watched at a distance. Better understanding helps in judging how to deal with him as an individual. In assessing mood it is not wise to take what he says at face value such as expression of feelings of weakness or helplessness. How he actually behaves may reveal indications of depression or perhaps laziness.

The practice of reality orientation which is often used with confused people is based on humanitarian values including respect for personal dignity (Holden and Woods, 1982). In attempting to rediscover the whole person and promote autonomy, decision making is encouraged in all suitable areas of life, and the environment designed to be as helpful as possible. People are offered the chance to be heard, although this means the listener may have to try and interpret without taking all such expressions of helplessness, at face value.

Attempts by a patient at what seems like attention-seeking behaviour for its own sake on a ward soon becomes like a cry of 'wolf' and tends to be ignored. An example of this is the patient who asks every passerby for a commode. This happens in some cases after the patient has wet the bed on a previous occasion and now feels extra anxious to avoid a repetition. Some patients might use this as a ploy just because they are immobile and unnaturally worried so that frequent urinating becomes an activity they focus on. An attempt to listen and understand can reveal a difficulty that could be resolved in part because proper attention has been given and the troublesome patient has been given a choice to behave otherwise encouraged by reassurance and some gentle discipline.

Privacy

In normal everyday private life people guard their right to avoid unwanted interference in their lives, invasion of modesty or public knowledge of behaviour as each wishes. When admitted to an institution this is one right that is hard to preserve to any extent. All health care staff through exposure to so many people risk becoming careless of others' feelings in this respect but patients could feel demeaned and upset if this is neglected.

Probably most patients accept some loss of privacy in hospital, at first in return for the reassurance of being in reliable care. Many of those who are very ill are beyond caring as are those who lose inhibition as part of mental illness. In all cases, however, attempts at preservation of dignity should be maintained in personal clothing, in discussion about their medical condition or social situation. It can be easy for a physiotherapist to forget how hurtful exposure of the body or personal social details might be. This is particularly so for an elderly person who has lived alone perhaps for more than 40 years, or equally for a woman from a country where she is used to being totally covered at all times. Staff should be sensitive to the patient's embarrassment at using an unlocked toilet because he needs assistance or a bath when people come and go past a half-opened door. Disturbing someone at a quiet activity such as reading, at prayer or a hobby should be done with caution and apology.

Attention to the caring team

If the patient is going to receive the optimum support from his family and he wants opportunity and permission to be as self reliant as possible, then they need to be put in the picture. The more dependent the patient is on physical help the harder it would be for him to maintain any areas of activity as he has to wait on another's convenient moment. The physiotherapist should be able to help by explaining and demonstrating how much he can safely do alone, no matter how slowly, and emphasize the importance for the patient himself to carry out even small tasks. It can be very frustrating for family members to allow this. If he is a wilful risk taker or lazy, conflict with the family may be modified. Explanation of the condition and listening to the family report of difficulties is even more important when the patient has mental illness. This would be offered by the doctor, but many practical problems on preserving areas of choice might be eased by discussion with a physiotherapist.

On a busy surgical ward where the patients are at all levels of activity and response it can be hard for the ward staff to know individuals or their difficulties in mobility. A physiotherapist can make a useful contribution to the management and recovery of a multiply disabled elderly patient simply by discovering how much he can do or needs to be helped and sharing it with the appropriate nurse. He can then be encouraged to do what is possible.

The physiotherapist needs to try to understand others' handling difficulties and be prepared to work out the best methods adapted for that member of staff and the patient. Jointly agreed methods and shared interest in the patient's independence will help to foster improved personal care. The physiotherapist might think he should undertake certain activities, even just washing his face, for reasons of physical well being as well as morale. Any such activities should be promoted with the co-operation of the nursing staff so that as many areas of independence in grooming or dressing may be perpetuated (See also Chapters 5 and 7.)

HOW IS IT DIFFERENT WITH OLDER PEOPLE?

If one of the tasks of a physiotherapist is to help a patient take some responsibility for his own recovery, or in maintenance of activity it is one that requires judgement on several counts. She needs to appreciate the social and psychological effects of long life, disability and relationships.

Social history

Many people who have grown up during this century and in this country have suffered multiple difficulties caused by widespread poverty, social inequalities, two World Wars and the Depression. Post-war prosperity and the Welfare State have improved material conditions, but for many, especially women, their lives have been lived against a background of hard work, poverty and loss. Some have also suffered racial discrimination. This will have differed according to individual histories, but affects expectations and attitudes of people in older age groups. Due to evictions, job loss and lack of control in the past, some people have a low level of expectation, assertiveness and standards of comfort. Others who have held positions of authority and maintained control over their lives and movement would have different attitudes, but based on a long term of experiences. Mark Abrams found in a survey of 1646 people aged over 65 that those living alone were more satisfied on all topics that were discussed than those living with others (Abrams, 1978). These topics included mobility difficulties, loneliness and life satisfaction. It could be assumed that the stimulus of being independent was an important reason. A great importance for those over 75 was placed on primary social relationships, but good health which was related to mobility was also ranked high in value for all. Money and travel were judged much less important.

How people cope with events of life depends on personality. A patient who has had plenty of experience is likely to have developed patterns of coping. Every conquest will have provided confidence for

39

the next time. He may not ever have been in hospital during his 80 years but there will have been other challenges. Alternatively, someone who has endured a lifetime of perceived low status, or lack of control over his life is unlikely to be assertive in old age, though he may be stoical or content with his lot. Admission to an institution could have been the culmination of a long struggle to be independent. Generalization is quite imprudent for there will be as many reactions as there are people, but coping with changes of environment is said to get harder. It can be surprising to younger physiotherapists, however, quite how well many older people respond to encouragement in self reliance. Compliance in the practice of home exercises if they have been well taught can be high. Feelings do not diminish in intensity with age. Grief at loss of friends, home, or even bladder control can be overwhelming. Equally, pleasure at compliments or true friendliness would be as heart warming as ever.

Disability

Illness such as polio or tuberculosis, or an injury early in life, leaves some individuals with permanent joint deformity or weakness which, although limiting activity, seems not to have prevented a fully participating life. Others manage to maintain independence in self care despite longstanding rheumatoid arthritis or a slowly developing multiple sclerosis. A further burden such as a joint sprain which might be of minor importance to most people, can deprive them of treasured activity. Shoulder pain for someone in a wheelchair or a fairly minor knee problem that prevents an already disabled person climbing into a bus could be a cruelly depriving impairment for either. Careful attention should be paid to help such people recover whichever independent activity they think is important.

Relationships

Long-term relationships within a family, whether between husband and wife or parent and child are likely to be in a set pattern for good or ill until sickness, death or change of dwelling has a marked effect on the extent of the strain. Whether it is good or unhappy, the physiotherapist cannot change this, but in promoting self reliance for the patient should be aware of the importance of the character of the relationship. The carer might raise a multitude of objections to the patient's being able or allowed to carry out certain activities. Another would be glad for him to try anything. It is likely that their relationship is more important than the state of dependence noted in hospital or when the therapist is in the house. A patient who is dependent is particularly vulnerable to family changes. Younger members may become unavailable to help because of work or children. If old friends and neighbours are important in the patient's life, it might be wondered how much he might lose by being away from his home for long days of treatment at the day hospital. An unneeded service no matter how fine will sap independence and is always wasteful. Not only that, but he might lose his friends as well.

3

Goal setting

Good practice in physiotherapy requires the establishment with each patient of agreed individual goals, both short and long term. Goals should be realistic, subject to on-going review, discussion and modification. A specific end result should be identified and priorities established.

WHAT IS GOAL SETTING?

For anyone who aspires to pass a test of physical prowess the aims are more or less obvious depending on the level of difficulty. If the test is running a race, the finishing post is set up and each competitor knows exactly how to get there and where he is going.

The process of patient care should also have momentum and a sense of direction. In the usual treatment system the patient comes to the physiotherapist, presents a problem, expects and is given the means of solution. An example of this could be a patient with a simple sprained ankle, no other ailments or social difficulties. The goals are obvious and on the face of it require no discussion. With treatment, patient and physiotherapist collaboration, swelling and pain are lessened speedily and the leg restored to full use. The problem was simple, the progress direct.

In learning an intricate gymnastic routine or to play a musical instrument the skilled procedure requires a complicated process involving stages of learning simple postures and movements. Once these are achieved plans are made to learn the more difficult sequence. Thus, over a period of training, a series of goals are aimed for, a new balance posture, a new piece of music, each depending on a previous success. The final result is a skilled sequence of movements that the pupil could not imagine at the outset. Final goals of treatment can also be difficult for the patient or even the therapist to see clearly at the outset. This may be due to the severity of a major accident or the interaction of many obstacles. After a short period in hospital it may be possible for the professional team to agree on a general aim of management, whether this be restoration of function or maintenance of activity and comfort. Also for people seen at home or as outpatients, a long-term general plan which will determine the manner and direction of treatment should be agreed fairly soon.

Goals should be realistic and be specific at each stage. As each problem is tackled progressively, with small intermediate objectives set and achieved by the agreed time, a realistic final goal will gradually become clearer. This process is achieved by collaborative team work including the patient. The sequence of rehabilitation is given a sense of direction and purpose. Even for a patient whose physical state does not improve, the overall aim of maintaining the status quo with maximal satisfaction to all concerned may still be facilitated by clearly stated goals with objectives that can be measured.

HOW IS IT DONE?

Identify realistic goals

The identification of suitable goals for management and treatment of a patient's difficulties begins with the examination and assessment followed by listing his problems and assets. This problem list will help to focus attention on priorities for action. Dr Partridge has given warning of the risks of seeing these too narrowly from the professional point of view. Her investigation of the patients' and physiotherapists' perception of progress after a stroke or wrist fracture revealed at the second enquiry only a 37% correlation of agreement between the two (Partridge, 1984). The reason for this appeared to be that patients viewed their main problems as restrictions in functional activity, whereas the physiotherapists had listed problems of performing movements in terms of clinical signs.

More importantly, in this study patients' and physiotherapists' perceptions of progress were at odds, the latter being more optimistic. Patients were said to be frustrated and complained that staff made unrealistic claims of progress. This is perfectly understandable when a physiotherapist takes pleasure in the early signs of

43

recovery although this has no immediate and obvious functional outcome. Agreement on aims and progress probably could have been resolved by explanation and discussion.

Goals aimed at motivating the patient must relate to the patient's problems. To begin this it would be essential to discover what the patient already knows and understands. The physiotherapist is then in a position to explain the implications of his condition, and through discussion and during the early treatment sessions help to balance his expectations and abilities.

Example: Mr Rust, aged 76, has over the previous six months become almost inactive following a fall in the garden after which he suffered some backache. He needs help to rise from his armchair and no longer goes to the bowling club.

Examination reveals some slowing of movements in his right limbs as compared to the left. He still complains of backache on standing up, and has a tendency to lurch backwards when walking around corners in the house. He talks vaguely of wanting to get to his greenhouse, but has not been out. His wife is apprehensive of his falling.

The tentative goals of husband and wife seem to be conflicting. The physiotherapist would be able to help Mr and Mrs Rust analyse the plus and minus factors, then propose a realistic overall aim, perhaps to help Mr Rust be more active. If he wishes to get to his greenhouse, then all sorts of intermediate stages will have to be gained such as rising easily from his chair, and controlling his balance while walking. This, of course, is likely to be facilitated with the help of an occupational therapist if fixed rails or furniture alterations are needed. It will be achieved largely through Mr Rust's efforts, with encouragement and treatment from others, but his motivation is essential. Sometimes this is aroused only when some achievement can be appreciated. When he has reached the greenhouse he may be ambitious enough to resume bowling.

It was noted in a Californian study of physiotherapists' age bias in setting goals for older patients, that those of the group who set more 'aggressive' goals had a more positive attitude towards ageing and the aged (Sharon, et al., 1986). It was thought that this finding possibly reflected an individualized approach to patients. Certainly if a therapist sets a lower than justifiable goal for an old patient, he, taking her views, may fail to achieve his potential.

Some patients, typically when desperate to be at home perhaps following a stroke, seem to be quite unrealistic and do not appreciate the limitations.

Example: Mrs Davison, hoping to return home soon after a third stroke might think she can walk quite safely enough using a wheeled walking frame. Unless the reason for spending time in exercises to improve her balance reactions, and the importance of her managing to turn, bend and cope with clothing in the toilet is explained, she might well become despondent at the delayed discharge. Once this intermediate goal is agreed, she is likely to concentrate and try harder.

Expectations of the outcome will be informed also by knowledge of the natural history of the condition with its associated prognosis. The classification formulated by Dr Partridge takes into account these broader issues against which the specific clinical history of the individual may be set (Partridge, 1980).

Group 1. Patients with soft tissue injuries and conditions will often be localized to one site, such as sprains, and tenosynovitis.

For these patients, since resolution is expected in time anyway, the effect of any therapeutic intervention relates to hastening recovery by relieving symptoms.

Group 2. Patients who have conditions which essentially require other management or treatment, physiotherapy forming only one part of the treatment programme and often relating to only one aspect of the patients' condition.

Patients who have fractures, who have undergone surgery or medical treatment for cardiac failure are examples in this group. Recovery is expected with correct management, but there would be the possibility of development of maladaptive practices.

Group 3. Patients with conditions which involve irreversible damage to or loss of body tissue, and therefore some lasting disability is expected.

Examples in this group are patients who have suffered a cerebrovascular accident, or had a limb amputated. There will be a wide range of outcome from minor lesions where a return to near-normal functioning is expected to those with major damage or loss which limits the extent of possible recovery.

45

Group 4. Patients in whom progressive deterioration is expected.

A large number of conditions seen by therapists come in this group, for example, motor neurone disease, osteoarthrosis and Parkinson's disease. For some patients the emphasis of treatment will be on localized relief of symptoms, but usually the aims will be more general and relate to regaining and maintaining levels of functioning ability.

In practice many patients fall into more than one category.

Example: Mr Burrows has had a fractured neck of femur and undergone surgery to fix this. In addition he has longstanding osteoarthrosis of one knee and a previous stroke.

Mr Burrows has been independently mobile in his house and garden prior to the accident. The fracture is fixed and is expected to heal well (Group 2). The osteoarthritic knee is swollen and painful due to damage caused at his fall (Groups 1 and 4). The effects of the stroke (Group 3) may be exacerbated by the recent events.

Set measurable conditions

Aim of management

The aim of management (rehabilitation to independence in daily activity within the house in Mr Burrow's case) would take all the factors mentioned above into consideration.

Intermediate goals

The intermediate goals are more specific and relate to the details of what each patient needs to achieve in his environment. These intermediate goals should be identified and recorded in definite terms as shown in Table 3.1 (see also Evaluation, p. 110).

Once these goals have been achieved and Mr Burrows has gone home, a further set of goals will be agreed, including his getting down the back steps to his workshop, perhaps. The goals should be understood by all concerned.

The goal conditions should be:

1. measurable
2. stated in exact terms, and
3. to what degree of success (see Table 3.1)

46

Table 3.1

Who will	Do what	Under what specific conditions	By which date
Mr Burrows will be able to	1. Get himself in/out of bed	Alone	30 July
	2. Stand up from an arm chair	17 in high, unaided	6 August
	3. Walk a distance of 20 feet	Using a walking frame	13 August
	4. Turn and sit down	Safely with supervision only	20 August

Most functional activities can be measured in terms of time or distance or frequency according to the important factors. For one patient it could be important that he be able to walk a certain distance, no matter how slowly. For another patient control of balance long enough to stand in the toilet could be a priority need. The degree of success is relevant to the level of stamina of the patient or helper. Too many failures would sap his meagre strength or increase the need for supervision. It might be decided that a low level of success is acceptable in view of his condition, and that a fit helper at home can cope with the situation. For reasons of encouraging morale the terms of each goal should be (a) simple, and (b) achievable.

To help the patient along it would assist to seek out quite small goals so that he can be motivated by success and thereby gain in self esteem. One person might aim to increase standing time by only a few seconds, to climb another step each time, or practice an easy exercise to a set prescription. In the case of a patient with a recent stroke for whom standing was laborious, it would be useful to set a certain date to achieve for sitting unsupported on a firm base since this might be accomplished fairly soon. For a patient who is depressed, or partly demented, it is also important to set easy goals in order to boost morale and that praise is given for actual achievement.

If the patient can suggest his own next step, even if it needs modification, that would be a morale booster also. A balance might have to be drawn between his expectation and ability, but the task probably would be a useful one. To be realistic in acknowledgement of the variability of human powers, each goal should be reached

47

three times before being considered won. It is likely, no matter how limited the goal, that the sense of achievement will be satisfying.

Objective steps

In planning the achievement of a goal there will be stages on the way. The scheme of treatment will be most useful if these are considered in terms of objective steps. These are based on the analysis of steps to recovery.

To achieve Mr Borrows' goal of standing unaided the objective steps will measure his progress in easy stages.

Objective steps – stated in terms of practical aims

Day 1. Mr Burrows to sit in a chair of appropriate height.

Day 10. Able to stand up with help of one person and to lean on a frame.

Day 20. Able to stand up with supervision of any member of staff plus frame for 20 s.

Day 25. As above with wife.

Day 30. Stand up – stand unaided 20 s plus wife's supervision.

What is being described is usually planned informally, and often in the physiotherapist's head. In a complicated or long-term case, however, it is helpful to all concerned if the plan is recorded in clear terms. For simplicity's sake it would often be sensible to have few written objective steps, perhaps only one or two at a time. When one is achieved, then the next can be planned. It is not always possible to predict very far ahead.

With experience a therapist will be able to forecast several weeks ahead in some cases. The system allows a basis for useful discussion, a means of learning, and of evaluating schemes of management by projected outcome, e.g. if the plan did not work, why not?

Full collaboration in goal setting may not be gained with a patient who is unable quite to understand, but as far as possible this should be sought. The goals should be set with the carers. Objective steps should be explained to the patient. With regular consistent attempts at practice, the goals may be perceived by the patient who would then collaborate more willingly.

For a patient in whom increased activity is not expected, maximal independence at quite a simple level might be the aim. The goal

Table 3.2

Subject	Task	Conditions	Review
Mr Chambers	Will stand up	At least twice daily	To be checked every month
	Walk to/from toilet or meal table	With one helper	

could be stated in specific terms related to the level of activity to be maintained. This might be a certain distance to be walked, its frequency and amount of support, or a list of self-care tasks such as hair combing or dressing (Table 3.2). He can then be pleased with what he can do, rather than lament at what he cannot do. Included in the list, as a reminder of the patient's state of well being, could be other occupations such as reading of newspapers, card games or knitting. If these are appreciated by the patient, but no longer pursued, the cause might be found to be remediable.

WHO NEEDS TO KNOW?

If the patient is going to be given real encouragement and help in achieving functional activity, all those who visit and help him need to know what he is aiming at. Inappropriate urging or even teasing to do more than is currently sensible may be discouraging, especially if every helper is making different demands. If everyone realizes a task is recently achieved, then praise is helpful and deserved. Everyone may share the credit for helping and pleasure at the patient's success.

The use of simple and clearly visible flow charts, or a star system can be useful to remind changing hospital ward or residential home care staff of the man's current activity and the next goal. A public display system might be of most use in a hospital where the change in patient's functional activity could be very slow. A system of symbols used to report a patient's difficulties and skills as described by therapists in Glasgow would lend itself to describing that patient's goals also (Richie and Lough, 1988). Without stated and dated goals referring to maintained ability, the effect of faulty memory and the onward rush of time, a sense of purpose and direction may be lost. When the patient is in hospital there may be conflicting goals or time expectations in the minds of different members of staff, the relatives, the neighbours, and the patient himself. If he is in a residential home, or his own home, there are fewer sources of opinion, but the conflict is none-the-less difficult to balance. There can be misunderstandings which discussion of goals in the context of long-term aims can help to resolve. It is not safe to assume agreement without ascertaining the other opinions. Doctors, wives or occupational therapists may have other goals and priorities.

There may be certain hidden goals that were best not made public knowledge, but generally, patient confidentiality is not breached by this system. Goals kept hidden are likely to be those related to patient behaviour when it might not be appropriate for him, or even a family member to know for fear of causing distress.

WHAT IF THE PATIENT SHOULD FAIL TO SUCCEED?

If the patient does not achieve any goal the first point to consider might be whether the difficulty had been identified accurately or whether the goal was, in fact, achievable. If the answer is yes, the next task is to examine various influences; external factors, the patient and the physiotherapist (see p. 139).

An external factor might be the failure of transport to the out-patients department so that treatment was less than had been planned, or new family circumstances; a move of house or illness of another member. The goal might have to be altered unless the problem is remediable.

The patient's condition can change, and so the whole situation will have to be re-assessed and goals negotiated. If the goal, in the opinion of the physiotherapist, should have been gained, perhaps the patient was apathetic, unwilling or had failed to understand. In any case there would be a need to discuss, re-negotiate or explain. It would be a waste of time just to plod on with unavailing treatment.

The alternative area of investigation is the physiotherapist's treatment. She would need to question among other things, her choice of technique, the tool for the job, her personal approach. Possible refinements of style, timing or frequency of exercise could be altered. The tools of electrical equipment, furniture, walking aids, games equipment could be considered. In one case if a patient does not accomplish a walk of a certain distance, re-examination might demonstrate the need for breakdown and re-acquisition of particular skills. He might need to spend more time just practising balance

Figure 3.1 What if the goal is not achieved?

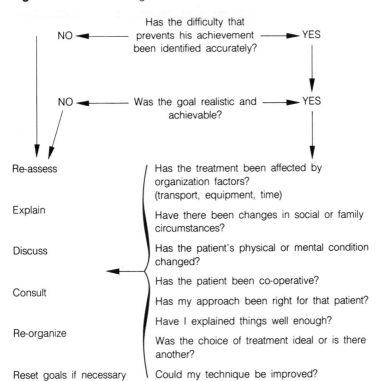

while standing. He might need to try a different, or even no walking aid. If the goal is the appropriate one, more specific advice can be sought from colleagues.

If it can be seen that a goal is not being achieved there may be reasons connected with the original assessment. The patient and physiotherapist may have too great an expectation of his progress or its speed. Perhaps the patient is in fact functioning at an appropriate level for his physical or mental strength, and no improvement could be expected.

In all these situations the physiotherapist can blame the patient, someone else, or go back a stage and re-examine the case, re-assess expectations, then come to some agreement with the patient and others concerned. The goal of increasing activity could be changed to one of maintenance for a time, then review. It is not sensible to keep putting the completion date off, leaving the patient striving (or not striving) for the wrong goal and all the carers at crossed

51

purposes. If the patient is at his full potential in one area of activity it could be useful to look sideways. In other words, if he cannot walk safely at home, agree that he continues to stand daily, but meanwhile explore other ways of employing his mind and time. In this way his maximal health, comfort and safety is maintained while nobody is worrying that he is not doing enough or too much (Figure 3.1).

HOW IS IT DIFFERENT WITH OLDER PATIENTS?

The process of goal setting is no different to that used with disabled children or younger adults. Appropriate aims are identified, goals may be agreed and target dates set. There are some different factors to be considered with elderly patients, such as different multiple pathology, life expectations, social features and psychological effects of long-endured disability.

Some older patients will have survived more than one illness or accident, which will have left residual effects. Goal setting may have to take into account troublesome degenerative joints, fading eyesight or deteriorating memory where these are evident. When conditions cause continued decline of faculties and activity due to general frailty or disease, so coping with these rather than recovery will have to be considered. Fortunately there is a large proportion of the population who seem to be amazing survivors and defy the commonly offered prognostications. Some make light of their disabilities, and in others the biological effects of ageing appear minimal.

Setting goals takes on a tentative quality when the patient's condition keeps changing, especially if he is likely to deteriorate grossly or die. In this situation the aim of management might be the maintenance of comfort or the optimizing of the individual's capability, but the intermediate goals could keep changing. At any time, he might be aiming to walk a certain distance, maintain his ability to feed himself or just sit in a chair in comfort. It is likely that a greater proportion of people over 70 than younger ones will be in this situation.

There are elderly people who depend to a large extent on social support systems, and often more than the individual realizes, especially if the intensity has grown slowly or if it has been gracefully given. If, however, the burden on relations or neighbours becomes suddenly greater, or has built up slowly almost to breaking point, their own health or circumstances alter, then the previously satisfactory regime may collapse. In certain cases a pause of a month or two is enough to allow those carers to appreciate the extent of their task enough to feel unable to continue. It is likely that family carers in this age group are also elderly and sometimes disabled. Plans for continuing at home or being discharged from hospital must take these factors into account.

Contemporaries, friends or siblings may well be in the same boat so far as health and activity go. Repeated news of illness or death of friends is not very encouraging. Repeated changes of dwelling can affect health adversely. Some of these contemporaries will not be optimistic about each others expectations. This will influence the outlook of someone who is considering the next stage of rehabilitation, or even the near future, and his chances of independence or contentment. Long-term ill health or disability has unpredictable influence on attitudes, and therefore goal planning, but a long history must be taken into account. Conversely, stable circumstances, close family ties, or possession of resilient personality will affect outlook. In situations where a goal seems to have to include a move from his own home, the loss of a licence to drive a car, or possibility of resuming a favourite activity, agreement between patient and therapists might be slow in coming. The physiotherapist, especially if perhaps only one-third of the patient's age, must realize when urging independence, all the multitude of influential memories and discomforts the older person may be coping with.

4

Treatment

The best results in treatment require the highest standards of physiotherapy and the sharing of some appropriate skills and knowledge with others involved with the patient. Teaching of the patient is of great importance followed by regular practice of an exercise with information on results.

WHAT DOES TREATMENT CONSIST OF?

Definition

The term treatment is limited for present purposes to the actual therapeutic activity that takes place during immediate contact between a physiotherapist and one or more patients. Treatment activity is often continued subsequently by the patient with or without help, but as a result of the advice offered during the contact period. It is distinct from other activities to do with an individual patient, such as examination, goal planning, talking with relatives and all the other tasks that may complete the overall management.

All physiotherapy can be described as consisting of 'natural methods based essentially on movement and manual therapy and on other physical agencies' (Williams, 1986a).

Teaching and motivation

With all treatment schemes the important components include teaching, of which motivating the patient is a part, and the selection of the appropriate modality for the focus of treatment. These are both factors in achieving both a satisfactory treatment result and patient compliance both at the time and in the future. If the patient understands the reason for his referral for physiotherapy, and the goals of the treatment, he is likely to appreciate the rationale behind the programme. For example, a patient with osteoarthrosis of the knees needs to know what his effort will achieve, possibly what the limitations are to achievement, and how he should look after his joints in future, in addition to receiving any specific symptom relief.

Teaching is not just telling, of course, but starts with motivating the patient to want to know the relevant facts before informing him about possible strategies to gain success.

The term motivation is difficult to define, but refers to the drive or desire to act in a certain way to achieve a certain end. The commonly used label of 'poorly motivated' implies a wilful decision by a patient to reject rehabilitation against the advice of the professional (Hesse and Campion, 1983). Poor motivation should be tackled as a problem to be resolved. The physiotherapist should listen to the patient, which includes watching for non-verbal signals, to try to identify his wishes. The rehabilitation setting can be unhelpful for some older patients if the pace of activity is too fast, for example. The sign of agitation or apathy may be noticed.

The motivation of a young athlete after an injury is seldom considered a problem, although achieving his compliance with treatment may be another matter. Most people after injury or temporary illness have adequate desire to resume previous activity, but enthusiasm for active treatment may not be so easy to stimulate in a patient with chronic disability, especially late in life. The possible reasons for this are outlined in the last section of this chapter.

Arousal of a patient's motivation by a physiotherapist requires her perception of his personality and needs. The special nature of physiotherapist–patient relationship has some features which can promote a patient's well being and thereby his motivation to try what she suggests. Compared to some other members of the team, a relatively large amount of time is spent in a face-to-face encounter which allows time for discussion and questions. The therapeutic effect of physical contact, whether during examination of a joint, the guiding of a movement, or in the conscious attempt to comfort is of immense importance in healing. The practical nature and immediacy of treatment which is conducted by the physiotherapist can be understood and appreciated as relevant by the patient. The patient can be and should be a participant in his therapy, not an onlooker (Pratt, 1978).

Ascertaining both what the patient understands and what he wants to know about his condition is important. Although this can often be done in a straightforward manner there are instances, such as in deteriorating or seriously disabling conditions where the therapist may have to spend time with the patient in order to discover the extent of his worries. A patient who has had a stroke may be confused and not able to understand that he has lost movement control. The therapist would have to use demonstration, careful handling techniques and explanations in order to avoid the patient becoming frustrated. These efforts may have to be repeated at intervals. Generally understood language should always be used rather than medical or physio-therapists' jargon. Sometimes it is sensible to check the patient's understanding in case a technical term has been used inadvertently.

The examination should have revealed the extent of medical, physical and psychological functioning so that realistic goals can be set. The expectations of the carers, both family and any nurses or care assistants should be examined. Small functional gains may not be valued highly by all staff, though they be all the patient desires. He may need an advocate to support him in his own resolve. All physio-therapy treatments require a certain amount of teaching and the compliance of the patient whether this be simple movement, use of transcutaneous nerve stimulation or a functional activity. Additionally there will be instruction on future health care for patient and/or carer.

After promotion of the motivation to learn and exchange of informa-tion, comes the rehearsal of the information or practice of activity. Learning styles vary according to individual's social background and personal attributes which the teacher should take into account. Some movements would be more easily learned if they are related to another familiar task. A reaching movement for example, could be likened to a household job. Information on care of degenerating joints might be linked by analogy to keeping a vintage car going.

Success in the patient's learning and activity depends on the skill of the teacher in providing clear verbal and/or manual instruction in the appropriate quantity for that individual. For example, if a patient needs to learn how to perform lumbar flexion as an exercise to relieve backache, he is usually given the reason first and encouraged to assume the starting position. Instruction on performance is given, each movement in sequence. Correct performance may be confirmed and mistakes corrected during the sequence. If the patient gets it wrong the teacher is at fault, perhaps just by being too hasty. In the attempt to improve walking style, the whole of the movement may be broken down into manageable stages, thus making success easier to achieve. There is nothing quite like success for promoting learning perhaps especially following the results of brain damage such as from a stroke.

56

For effective movement learning it has been demonstrated that feedback should be immediate. A trial conducted on experienced golfers who were trying to improve their putting style and being given immediate feedback information on head and body movements, showed a statistically significant increase in the number of putts holed (Simek and Brown, 1978). Comments to a patient should be specific as well as timely.

Just the demonstration of a technique or activity to a carer or patient is inadequate for learning. That person has to perform that same act with guidance and encouragement. As preparation or on occasions when performance of a manoeuvre is impracticable, the learner can absorb some of the information by telling the physiotherapist what to do stage by stage. The latter must avoid anticipating the next movement, of course.

Although feedback on performance should be generous at first, the patient has to learn to assess and correct his own performance. It has been shown during a trial of women aged 75–85 who were learning a balance skill, that mental practice, including the imagined feel of that movement performed perfectly, improved the performance more than 100% (Fansler, Poff and Shephard, 1985). Although this technique was more effective with some people than others, it was surmised that the aptitudes of clear imagination and self control would promote automatic self monitoring via the central nervous system. This technique might be attempted with alert patients who would be trying to improve walking skills following a mild stroke.

An effective deterrent to learning is stress on the learner's part. This can be compared to frequent interjections while one is memorizing a poem or even carrying out a simple task that requires concentration. (Perhaps some patients who find it difficult should be allowed to walk undistracted by others' movement or conversation.) Stress is also caused by pain, failure or even fear of failure. The physiotherapist must always try to promote trust by knowing how much stress the patient can take and asking for the possible in activity. She should never give the impression she is not sure of what she is doing (Wagstaff, 1982).

For establishment of a new skill, or recovery of an impaired one, practice sessions must be discussed and arranged. Success in learning is also affected by a patient's failure to retain the information, but good teaching will help to achieve his potential, especially if tasks are kept simple and repetition is frequent. Successful outcome will depend to some extent on the skill of the physiotherapist identifying realistic goals.

Aims of treatment and areas of apparent overlap

The specific treatment will be selected from a range of options. Since physiotherapy is usually directed to signs, symptoms and problems rather than root causes of illness the aims often include the following:

Relief of pain
Clearance of airways
Re-education and support of good posture
Stretching or loosening of soft tissues that limit movement
Strengthening of muscles
Control of abnormal muscle tone/re-education of normal movement
Stimulus of sensory appreciation and perceptive ability
Maintenance of skin and soft tissue integrity
Recovery or re-education of appropriate functional activities
Helping the patient to cope with disability
Continence of urine
Provision or supervision of the use and condition of aids and appliances
Prevention of maladaptive practices and postures
Reality orientation
Promotion of general fitness

The final goal of treatment is usually to improve or restore functional ability.

In some straightforward cases a simple modality will achieve the goal, for example in the relief of pain arising from a capsulitis of a glenohumeral joint on the non-dominant arm that may disturb sleep but not impair daily activity. Treatments for relief of activity-limiting pain in a knee may involve several modalities, for example, ice pack with specific and general exercise, followed by advice on care of the joint.

Sometimes a single measure will help to achieve several goals. The aim of guided or assisted standing following a stroke may be for the purposes of re-education of posture, normal muscle tone, balance, stimulus of sensation, maintenance of skin integrity as well as for reasons of physical health and patient morale.

It is important to ensure that exercise has an obvious practical purpose. The patient will probably comply with exercise for a stiff shoulder or unreliable balance if the outcome is being able to manage his dressing more efficiently. As mentioned before, treatment takes place both during the contact time and subsequently as a result of the teaching and advice. The outcome of an exercise that has a practical purpose is likely to be noticed when the patient is on his own.

Some functional activity that in physiotherapy is either part of re-education or practice for confidence, stamina or skill seems to overlap with other professionals' responsibilities (an occupational therapist or a nurse) (see pp. 145–6).

Observation of a patient drinking a cup of tea, dressing, or the assisting of someone in the toilet is part of physiotherapy when professional knowledge and skill may be needed to help achieve function. Analysis of the activity could be made; posture, balance, movement co-ordination and apparent anxiety level for example. This enables a specific choice of exercise to improve that function should it be necessary. Who is responsible for supervision of practice and maintenance of skills is sometimes a matter for discussion with other carers, whether in hospital or home.

Apart from the value of collaboration with the caring team in these practical tasks, and demonstrating the link up to the patient, useful observations can be made on how the patient manages in his customary setting, or perhaps how other carers see his difficulties or try to help. These observations will complement those made during formal treatment sessions. Getting off the customary hard plinth in a department may require some effort by a patient. The same procedure in the early morning complicated by stiffness, bedclothes, a soft mattress and haste to be somewhere else is likely to be more difficult. This is an argument for physiotherapists to be on a hospital ward for at least some early morning or evening sessions. Patients who are trying to recover independence in self care or mobility often need minimum but appropriate (i.e. not too much or too little) help. A physiotherapist who knows the patient's capability should offer to demonstrate this to others.

Difficulties can arise when care and treatment is shared between several professionals and there is uncertainty about others' aims and responsibilities. The 'grey' areas of overlap tasks, albeit with different purposes in care, must be discussed. Handling methods and expectations of the patient's capabilities must be agreed.

Ideally, all hospital ward staff should co-operate in promoting a patient's maximal independence on the basis of up-to-date shared information (Chapters 3 and 5). All functional activity practice, once the patient is judged able, can be supervised by any member of the ward staff or home carers. It will probably be up to the physio-therapist on the basis of regular assessment to make suggestions

59

about increasing or even reducing the demands made on the patient.

An elderly patient's ability may fluctuate or alter between early morning, mid-day and evening. In order to stimulate a realistic discussion with nursing staff or for accurate assessment for discharge home, knowledge of this performance variability is useful.

WHERE DO I START?

Reason for referral

When a patient presents with a new and obvious or troublesome problem with clear signs and symptoms the answer to this question is straightforward. After simple soft tissue trauma causing pain and swelling, the aftermath of cold orthopaedic surgery without complication, or recent chest infection, the immediate need or goal may be obvious. The problem list will help set priorities.

When the patient is disabled and in his own home, early attention will also have to be given to the carer's concerns. The physiotherapist may on the first visit help the carer in coping with essential daily tasks such as assisted transfer to a commode or the changing of bed linen, in addition to treatment of the patient's signs and symptoms.

In the case of a patient with multiple or gradually acquired impairment there may not be obvious or immediate priorities for attention. Assessment leading to problem identification, should reveal a starting point in the setting of short-term goals with the patient.

Example: Mr Artis, unable to rise from his chair with his swollen ulcerated legs, knees stiffened additionally by osteoarthrosis and one painful shoulder, may be keen 'just to walk'. Initial treatment may, however, need to be given for his leg oedema, improvement of leg muscle tone, shoulder pain, as well as doing something about chair height and shoes. If the man habitually wore only loose slippers due to swollen feet or his inability to tie laces, some other simply fastened boots might be obtained. It might have been possible for him to waddle a short distance having been hoisted to his feet, but that would not be of much real value unless he were enabled to get up and down by himself.

Maintenance of benefit

If benefit from treatment is to be retained, measures to perpetuate the effect should be undertaken in the early stages. Postural support for a painful joint is essential or the good effect of exercise or electrical treatment will be lost. Patients seldom appreciate this nor how simple adaptations to furniture may be achieved. As in the case of Mr Artis, efforts to rise from too low a sitting position are either unnecessarily painful or strenuous. Selection of a higher chair, or raising the chair seat by means of a folded blanket, for example, would ease his standing up. Back or hip ache which is present while sitting is often eased by good posture when it is firmly supported by appropriate padding, in most cases with spine straight or with a lumbar lordosis and hips near 90 degrees of flexion.

In the case of a patient with a chest infection, adequate air entry and efficient ability to cough is continued by well-placed pillows in bed or the choice of an appropriate chair supporting a straight thoracic spine, both during and following treatment.

If the stroke patient is to achieve purposeful and adaptable movements, it is important to pay attention early in rehabilitation to the patient's exact and symmetrical posture. This can only be continued if the family and professionals work together. Early on in the treatment programme it is often useful to come to some common agreement with the other carers on both purposes and frequency of treatment. This will confirm the patient's responsibility to do something on his own when this is possible (Chapter 3).

Common problems in treatment of elderly patients

Four of the problems in caring for elderly patients which have been identified as 'Giants of Geriatrics' are instability, incontinence, immobility and intellectual failure, to which depression can be added. In some patients when these are severe they are features to be taken into account in discussing with carers how best to cope. A physiotherapist may be able to offer advice and skills on handling or maintenance of physical mobility. At an earlier stage there may be scope for amelioration of these difficulties.

Instability

Lack of balance control, though variable between individuals

61

increases linearly with age as many studies have shown (e.g. Overstall et al.,1978). The chief risk of instability is falls, and the outcome of falls is not only fractures but the restriction of activity which may follow. This appears to be a factor which aggravates and accelerates the effects of ageing (Vellas and Cayla, 1987). In this study the outcome of falls and the result of the fear of falling resulted in failure of those people thereafter to visit friends (11%) among other losses.

Falls can be caused by a multitude of risks such as multi-pathology, multiple symptoms and multi-pharmacy. These factors include muscle wasting, debility, cardiovascular insufficiency, loss of visual acuity, dementia and antihypertensive drugs. Very often, however, there is an accumulation of non-specific, subclinical changes (Isaacs, 1985).

Despite all difficulties there is often scope for physiotherapy to improve the patient's capability by improving his general fitness, balance reactions and confidence. Anxiety gives rise to general muscle tension, thus reducing the body flexibility which is necessary for normal equilibrium and righting reactions. Re-education and practice of these movements in safe surroundings can help gradually in achieving optimal relaxation and confidence. Walking aids may be necessary, but can often increase general muscle tone inappropriately, disturb posture and prevent a natural walking pattern. Additional help may be gained by improving eyesight (correct and clean spectacles), diet and opportunities for social contact where these are necessary.

Gross instability of posture and movement is caused by damage to brain or spinal cord. The individual's awareness of his physical state is distorted by abnormal muscle tone, sensation and altered perception which would hamper his own attempts to recover control. Even in mild cases of polyneuritis or cervical cord damage for example, guidance by a physiotherapist would be required to facilitate and re-educate balance reactions to achieve optimum results. For patients after a stroke or other brain damage, the neurodevelopmental treatment (Bobath) approach is appropriate at any age in helping them relearn management of their own bodies again. The patients are guided in recovery of mobility as well as stability in the trunk which allows a better balance of tone. This assists in regaining an easier and more efficient use of the limbs. The principles have been described with reference to the 'geriatric stroke patient' by Bohman (1987) but practice of these techniques of analysis and handling require direct and practical teaching for best results.

Another sort of instability is that arising in joints affected by degenerative disease. Laxity in joint ligaments and synovial membranes with weakening of the supporting muscles leads to alteration of the biomechanical efficiency. Some osteoarthritic knees become grossly deformed in a valgus position and very insecure when bearing weight. Rheumatoid arthritis affecting neck and arm joints in some patients can render the limbs quite floppy. In some patients tendons rupture rather readily especially at the shoulder and metacarpo-phalangeal joints. Physiotherapy treatment for any of these includes advice in the early days of the condition in 'joint sparing' techniques to minimize joint damage. Splinting is sometimes necessary.

Incontinence

Failure to control the flow of urine before reaching a suitable recep-tacle is an embarrassing complication and not unknown for a person of any age. There are many causes which can be alleviated as a result of methodical investigation, but the symptom is often unreported by the individual due partly to social taboos on discussing the subject and resulting lack of awareness that anything can be done to relieve matters. Complications are added in older people due to the attitudes of others who use incontinence of urine or faeces as an excuse for blame. With attitudes of therapeutic positiveness, know-ledge of causes and sensitivity to the patient's feelings, much can be done to achieve continence and enlighten public social attitudes (Stewart, 1980).

The range of causes of incontinence in elderly people includes those of internal origin such as pathology or psychology and external features of the environment. The first stage in treatment is to discover which of these is causing the problem. The physiotherapist may be one of the first people with whom the patient may discuss any difficulty of control because activity such as coughing or walk-ing provokes it. At what can be a relatively simple level of remedy, incontinence may be caused just because the person is unable to walk to the lavatory in time or cope with undressing when arrived, or sit down easily on a low seat. Both occupational and physiotherapists have a contribution to make in improving the patient's mobility, removable clothing, and access to the toilet.

Noticeable onset of urinary incontinence may be caused by feverish illness, drugs, social change, or even the stress of inter-action. Unconsciously expressed resentment between a carer and an old person who feels 'babied', can be a cause of bed wetting. This situation requires investigation into the patient's pre-morbid personality and sympathetic understanding of the interpersonal dynamics to determine the real cause (Thompson, 1980).

The physiotherapist may have a contribution to make in promotion of the patient's physical independence. If bladder training is being undertaken by the nursing team, then collaboration with the time-tabled bladder emptying must be ensured, and maximum effort made to maintain the patient's self respect (Shepherd, Blannin and Smart, 1980). Out in the world of activity also, the shame endured at this loss of control in self care can be a true handicap so should be tackled with sympathy and understanding.

Intellectual failure

The two major areas of mental disorder for elderly people are those whose illness is of organic origin (dementia, toxic confusion, neuro-logical conditions) and those with psychiatric illness (depression, anxiety states). In some cases both varieties are present, depression resulting from organic illness for example.

Of all chronic syndromes perhaps none is feared more than the loss of memory and cognitive function that is the hallmark of demen-tia. Studies reveal a high incidence in people aged over 70 years. A recent broadly based survey showed marked impairment of 4.5% of this age group with approximately equal number in institutions and at home. The total including the mildly impaired was assumed to be 8% (Clarke, Lowry and Clarke, 1986). The prevalence of marked impairment increased sixfold between the group aged 75–79 and those over 85 years (4%–22.3%) but of course that still leaves 77.7% with mild or no impairment of cognitive function in the latter group. Nevertheless, the burden to families of members who because of illness are unpredictable or aggressive and immobile, and indeed to that person himself, is immense.

The problems for the patient and physiotherapist that arise with cognitive impairment, in addition to signs and symptoms of Parkin-son's disease, multiple cerebral infarcts, or acute chest infection for example, affect the conduct of treatment rather than the overall aims. Nearly all patients with chronic brain failure present problems of mobility and contractures, including those with Alzheimer's disease rather later in their career.

It has been suggested that the prospect of caring for confused elderly people arouses feelings of anxiety and dread or pity in the therapist that are less common when dealing with purely physical disability. Lack of predictability in the patient's day-to-day responses and the loss of personality can present a challenge to maintaining a sense of purpose in the therapist (Davis, 1986). Goals of care have

64

to be focused on maintaining as high a quality of physical and mental life with support of spiritual life as long as possible. Mutual encouragement of the professional team is helpful as well as knowledge of others' experience in the use of helpful techniques in communication, teaching and physical handling. (See also Involvement of carers, p. 78.)

An important feature of achieving movement in patients with dementia is the gaining of a response which equals success no matter how small and even if it is assisted. New mobility then must be repeated to reinforce the memory. Sometimes non-verbal cues are better than words in provoking a response such as a series of chairs to walk to. A technique such as backward chaining can help in relearning a sequence of movements as is involved in turning to sit on a chair. The movements are learned in reverse order. In this way the exercise is finished with a successful outcome (Brown and Frith, 1986). If concentration is poor and brief, treatment should be conducted frequently but for very short periods. All staff in institutions should try to be consistent in requests, for example in the use of a walking aid or in the routine of walks to a meal table. This is one episode when physiotherapists can help and encourage other staff as well as be obviously useful.

Physical handling of a person who is muddled by another sense of reality has to be particularly careful so it can be interpreted by that person as being comforting. The confused patient should never be approached suddenly or from behind, but visibly. The use of music and rhythm in achieving movement whether actively or passively can be very helpful. In exercise groups physiotherapist and helpers try to get everyone to their feet, especially those who habitually sit or walk very seldom. Even those normally unresponsive may respond by movement to rhythm which can be assisted by the therapist (Hare, 1986).

Immobility

This term of 'immobile' by which patients are labelled by hospital staff is usually an exaggeration. It does not mean motionless but describes a state somewhere below the ideal level of full activity. Patients tend also to report 'I can't walk', meaning 'I can't walk outside as far as I should like'. Nevertheless even without being rendered motionless (which does occur for example with advanced Parkinson's disease) the state of relative immobility is certainly common.

65

Table 4.1 Some causes of 'immobility'

Joint stiffness/arthrodesis	Fear
Increased muscle tone	Pain
Weakness/debility	Depression
Oedema of legs	Apathy
Dyspnoea	Habitual laziness
Low furniture	Anxiety
Drug induced	

The label is usually given to one whose disability renders him unable to move about, not even a single joint. The causes are many and sometimes in one individual, multiple (Table 4.1). The table is in part a repetition of an earlier list (see 'Aims of treatment') and indicates why the physiotherapist is so often called in to try to improve matters.

For some patients the level of 'mobility' might vary from day to day, morn to eve or according to who is watching. Most physiotherapists will meet a situation where another helper will report that 'he won't do it for me'. It is not always 'won't', since it can be remedied by quite simple advice on technique of movement or choice of support.

When the cause has been discovered it may be partly or satisfactorily remediable. Sometimes much ingenuity and persistence are required and shown by elderly patients who want to get about. With the help of occupational therapists and physiotherapists using imagination and perhaps the provision of just the right aid few need be altogether chair-bound.

Even the unfortunate few will need to be moved from one chair to another or lavatory. If a method can be devised to enable them to assist in the transfers by taking some weight through their arms or legs, much strain on patients and helpers will be saved.

Depression

This is a major psychiatric illness of old age and often more entrenched than in younger persons. Among the environmental factors that lead to depression are the effects of ageing, reduced status and control, bereavement and illness. In severe cases, signs of dementia may be present, but intellectual failure is not a common effect of most depressions. The problems can be those of the physical illness that make a greater than ordinary impact on the patient's awareness, especially pain and loss of strength. In older people the added load of work after the death of one of a couple, places the bereaved under unusual physical strain which can be very disheartening. The therapist should be alert to patients' reports of difficulties even in minor tasks like cooking or bringing in the coal (Hare, 1985).

Other effects of depression include stooping posture, constant muscle tension, debility and weakness as a result of failure in self care, accidents or falls. Regular exercise is of great value starting at an easy level and progressing very slowly while being well within the patient's capacity. Poor posture and muscle tension in the long term lead to pain which may be counteracted by posture analysis and correction, with practice of relaxation techniques.

Challenges for the physiotherapist in treating the depressed patient arise in the need for exercising patience and empathy with the patient's recital of worries and misgivings. Sometimes the former will encounter hostility; more often a discouraging lack of positive motivation. Physical methods, however, have a real part to play in treatment of mental as well as physical illness and this knowledge can help provide encouragement to the therapist.

HOW DO WE CONTINUE?

Evaluation of effect

Treatments may be changed, adapted or ceased as seems best for the patient. Similarly, as goals are achieved new ones are tackled. Throughout the course of treatment patient records should be kept with record of outcome. In order to determine which modality is being effective, especially in pain relief, where it is notoriously hard to remember, the patient's important signs should be tested each time both immediately before and after treatment and enquiry made about the result several hours later. If even simple records are being kept of outcome, then no restorative or maintenance treatment need be pursued wastefully or in ignorance.

In some cases it is not easy to determine whether treatment is having an effect on maintaining function. At that stage some measurement may be taken and treatment stopped until the appointment for review.

The pursuit of treatment for its own sake is both misguided and misleading and the patient's expectations will be built on sand.

67

He will be unrealistic about his own potential and the eventual and inevitable cessation of 'treatment' will be interpreted by him as evidence that he cannot be cured. (Hawker, 1975)

Homework

If the patient is required to practise an exercise on his own, or adopt certain postures, postural drainage or an efficient sitting position, for example, the procedure should be made clear to him. This may be facilitated by demonstration and practice schedules or charts of simple instruction.

It has been found that patients remember scarcely half of what they are told by physicians (Ley, 1972) but this proportion is improved if:

1. the patient writes the information down
2. important information is given first
3. the advice is specific

Compliance in exercise programmes is said to be higher if the exercisers achieve their own goals and receive family support (Ice, 1985).

If advice amounts to more than a simple item it is therefore a sensible precaution to offer it to a patient in writing and/or picture form, checking that he can see, read and comprehend. If this is written to his own choice of words, understanding is promoted. It is usually wise to suggest only one exercise at first, adding others when the performance is checked and outcome known. Practice time and frequency should be agreed. The other form of practice monitoring without a physiotherapist is by the substitution of a trained helper who knows exactly what is expected, and who can provide moral and physical support as required, keeping the physiotherapist informed of changes in the patient.

When maximal restoration of ability has been achieved, or whatever the next goal had been, patients are discharged from hospital or community care. Treatment does not continue except for planned review. Ideally, discharge should be planned and agreed so that the patient maintains his confidence. In some cases patients are given a name and telephone number either of the hospital or community physiotherapist who may be contacted in cases of need.

Long-term care

When the patient seems to have recovered his potential for activity but has to remain in hospital, the next stage of management could be called long-term care. This may begin quite soon after admission if it is considered no gain could realistically be aimed for, or perhaps after six to nine months following a dense stroke after which the patient has had little resolution or does not respond to rehabilitation.

Although active rehabilitation may have ceased there is still a role for physiotherapy in helping a patient maintain his maximal activity and comfort, as well as help in the prevention of secondary complications caused by recumbency. This may just be an advisory and collaborative role with nurses about appropriate furniture, footwear or methods of assisted transfer from a chair. If the patient needs special help in walking or standing, physical help or extra encouragement, then somebody from the department, physiotherapist or helper, may be considered best to carry out this task. The value of standing, if at all possible for a few minutes daily needs to be explained to each new member of staff. The beneficial effects on breathing, digestion, elimination and bone structure are not always realized, even if the boost to morale of having his head at normal height is appreciated by the patient.

It is often more difficult to ensure continued activity in an old peoples' home where there are other priorities and few staff, even if the recipient of help is keen. The chief focus of attention must often be in helping the care staff to be aware of the importance of maintaining older peoples' independence. Careful teaching may have to be given about certain individuals especially after return or at first arrival from hospital. 'What you don't use you lose' is particularly evident in the first few days, especially if the new resident lacks confidence and the staff are unaware of his activity level. Individual treatment may be given to a patient in a residential home following a limb injury for example, as if he were in his own home. More often and quite as importantly is the general 'treatment' provided by advice to the care staff on appropriate methods of helping residents, choice of chairs and conducting activity classes. This has been outlined by Helen Ransome (1980) in describing the physiotherapy service to homes for the elderly in Greenwich.

Whatever the level of ability, whether it be getting off a chair or dressing, it can be lessened due to loss of strength and will. In practice, when movements are painful it is often difficult to decide

69

whether it is worth putting the patient through a lot of discomfort thus causing misery or resentment. A patient who has unsteady walking causes concern to some carers. These feelings when conveyed to the patient may affect his confidence. A realistic alternative activity to maintain health and leg strength could be standing by a fixed support, and 'walking' on the spot.

Physiotherapists have to be aware of the dangers of assessing elderly patients at one point in time and thus categorizing them for life. All patients with delayed recovery or at risk of losing functional ability must be kept constantly under review. Many are slow starters, but many given an interesting and stimulating environment and a positive attitude on the part of personnel involved, may discover a sense of volition and purpose (Hawker, 1975).

Other forms of promoting mental and physical activity are often shared by other disciplines – nurses, occupational therapists, leaders of exercise classes, and a variety of therapists using music, painting, reminiscence or craft as the medium. Where these life-enhancing facilitators are available, the role of the physiotherapist may be in encouraging or advising the professionals about an individual's capability or perhaps in collaborating in partnership.

HOW IS IT DIFFERENT WITH OLDER PATIENTS?

The need for a difference in treatment of many elderly patients with simple or single problems may seem slight, but there has to be a conscious sensitivity of approach by the therapist and awareness of the need to adapt techniques as necessary. Some of the reasons are the same as outlined in Chapter 1.

Differences in style and intensity may be required in the following aspects of treatment:

Active movement
Passive movement
Use of ice or electrical treatment
Personal approach
Adjustment to social factors
Length of session and frequency of practice
Compromises due to multipathology
Involvement of carers
Health education

70

Active movement

On the part of many elderly patients there will be expectations with respect to exercise levels that will be considered quite low by inexperienced physiotherapists. These people have adjusted to the normal ageing effects on muscles, joints and the cardiovascular system. Many, of course, will be less fit than they might be due to inadequate exercise, or obesity.

Cardiac stroke volume is less well sustained than in a young person (Shephard, 1985). For this reason exercise that would require prolonged or intense effort is not recommended, perhaps should not be necessary and might endanger life. In each case, with knowledge of the state of the heart and testing of exercise tolerance, the right level for each person can be confidently urged. For people who are functioning at less than their potential level of activity, practice, with guidance and encouragement can improve their current state. Activity at a low mechanical efficiency of effort and with adequate rest is suitable as well as safe. Repetition and a graduated programme will achieve the effect.

Muscle activity is dependent not only on the heart, but on good oxygen intake which in very old people is affected by reduced functional capacity and alveolar surface area of the lungs. This is due to fibrosing of connective tissue in the lungs, respiratory muscles and associated joints, perhaps in some by a kyphotic dorsal spine. Stiff joints and poor co-ordination, apart from other disability, increase oxygen need. Additionally, circulation time is prolonged by 33% at the age of 80 and myocardial contractibility is diminished. This should alert the therapist to be sensible in her demands of patient activity, especially strenuous movements such as walking with a leg encased in plaster or propelling a wheelchair.

There is a relative loss of muscle strength with age. Counts of large muscle fibres in active 70-year-old people revealed an average loss of 25% as compared with young adults. Tests of the strength of knee extension in subjects aged between 70 and 86 years showed a loss of 45% (Vandervoort et al., 1986). Although the muscle power of most people aged over 70 would be less than a young adult, for one of either age existing power can be increased by exercise.

Patients who have suffered sudden loss of function due to a stroke, illness or accident are likely to achieve less than their expectations because the reality of illness is hard to comprehend. Recovery at any age from a chest infection or operation and return to normal activity,

71

though usually longer than the individual expects, lengthens with the years. Old age narrows the range of adaptability to the effect of illness. Normally the loss of resulting function is gradual so people adjust their daily activities. It is the reserve capacity that is diminished.

Muscle strength that has been lost due to pain through damage, swelling, infection, debility or recoverable illness will return if these conditions can be reversed and careful rehabilitation activities are undertaken. Adequate help and stimulus will be required if the person's functional capacity has dropped below the level of being able to make a start, for example, to get up from a chair. In addition to the provision or adaptation of furniture to facilitate this process, exercise for the anti-gravity muscles either unresisted or against gravity alone is usually adequate.

Resistance to movement provided by weight lifting or other pressure can be harmful to joints with degenerative disease, compressing the surfaces unnecessarily severely and causing pain. Resistance can be added more safely in this situation by the use of rhythmic stabilization in the manner of proprioceptive neuromuscular facilitation and is less likely to provoke pain. Simpler alternative means include the use of increasing the time the muscle contraction is held, or the number of repetitions. The effectiveness of the combined educational programme with simple quadriceps contractions, in improving the function and reducing pain levels in patients with osteoarthrosis of the knee has been demonstrated (Adler, 1985).

Passive movement

Stretching of soft tissue around joints has to be undertaken with care in testing the existing limits. Even joints not apparently affected by degenerative disease or previous damage are likely to stiffen in old age with loss of elasticity in the connective tissue. The proportion of collagen increases and the tissue may even become calcified.

Some joints seem to be particularly susceptible to loss of range of movement, perhaps due to a previous inflammatory episode or damage, combined with habitual inactivity or daily movement that no longer includes a full stretch in all directions. Loss of shoulder range, especially elevation, is common, as is extension of hip and knee joints when they have undergone some degeneration. The patient may not have been aware or concerned. Passive movement will reveal by the quality of the end-feel whether any increase is likely to be gained by passive measures. If it is a hard end-feel, physiotherapy is unlikely to redeem matters. Passive stretching even with serial plasters is very seldom satisfactory due to the quality of connective tissue (mentioned above), apart from the other complications that would be provoked. Active means of prevention while it is still possible is preferable.

Temporary loss of range is not uncommon due to the factors of a degenerated joint; damage or inflammation, with general immobility, or spasticity. The joints are commonly painful when moved which causes extra muscle spasm. They become fixed unless measures can be undertaken to relieve the symptom. The customary remedies of pain relief measures, including support, muscle contraction and movement need to be modified with reference to connective tissue changes in skin, muscle and joint capsule. This requires prompt action before the joints become fixed. The use of a long inflatable boot with an intermittent air pressure pump may be worth trying for an immobile patient with a semi-flexed knee.

If serial splinting or prolonged traction are to be used to stretch soft tissues, frequent inspection of the part undergoing strain or pressure should be made. For reasons of diminished circulation, thinly covered bony points, muscle wasting or poor sensory awareness the skin covering may break. Skin is particularly vulnerable to shearing strain (Fernandez, 1987). The secondary complications of pressure sores, poor respiration, constipation, and lowered morale arise if this treatment requires the patient to be in bed. For these reasons, prolonged and constant bed rest is to be avoided. Even short periods out of bed each day and some activity should be encouraged. If the patient is unable to stand easily, the physiotherapist would need to check the range of movement in joints that might stiffen. She should be prepared to offer advice and demonstration to encourage other carers to share this task, especially if the patient is at home. The patient who is at risk of developing contractures is very likely to have been inactive so in need of special vigilance, with promotion of his maximal activity and frequent change of posture.

Passive joint mobilization whether for pain or stiffness is not contra-indicated, but should be undertaken with awareness of the likely current potential passive range and state of joint surfaces. Mobilization at grades IV and V (Maitland, 1977) are seldom indicated. Mobilization at a lower grade for pain will not be fully effective in an arthritic joint if the tissues, including mechano-receptor neurones, have degenerated, and this reduces the inhibitory effect on dorsal horn pain gate mechanism (Grieve, 1980).

The vigour of passive treatment given to assist coughing and clearance of lung secretions should be tempered by the realization that ribs might be brittle as well as tender. The incidence of osteoporosis in post-menopausal women is said to be among the most common clinical disorders of bone. The loss of trabecular bone and thinning of the cortices causes a steep rise in fracture incidence after the age of about 60 years (Ayalon *et al.*, 1987).

Ice and electrical treatment

Any treatment that requires the patient's co-operation and reporting of perceived intensity would be contra-indicated if the skin sensation seems deficient, if the patient is confused, has a poor short-term memory, or for other reasons is unable to communicate adequately. Sensation may be diminished for pathological reasons such as neuropathies, stroke or damage to sensory nerves at spinal nerve root level. This difficulty is more likely to be present in any older patient, but not of course certain. Some elderly people have acquired deafness so care must be taken that instructions are understood. Marked confusion would render such a patient unable to receive electrical treatment that could not be monitored by someone else. An electrical heat pad is probably a safe heat source.

The use of ice is seldom contra-indicated unless the patient has a problem with the circulatory system such as Raynaud's disease. Indeed it is perhaps the first choice of treatment to relieve pain of superficial soft tissue inflammation. Protection for sensitive skin is sometimes advisable but application of melting ice in a polythene bag or damp towel is usually safe. It should not be left in place longer than about 5–10 minutes for risk of over-cooling the area.

Personal approach

On each encounter with a new patient, the physiotherapist would introduce herself by name, and when necessary explain her role. The style of approach should be adapted to suit the occasion and the listener, but there are particular considerations with respect to older people. The reasons are to do with changes in sight or hearing, perceived status and common psychological traits. Many feel anxious in strange places, at confronting new people and about unexplained signs and symptoms in their own bodies. This may be exaggerated if hearing is poor so that the usual reassuring remarks made while facing away from the patient are unheard. If visual impairment renders the surroundings, labels, and even faces unrecognizable, especially for one who has been transported thither without explanation, this can give rise to great anxiety. Despite great differences in individuals, many hold themselves in low esteem, possibly due to experiences in the past of being dominated by circumstances.

For these reasons the physiotherapist needs to be especially positive but considerate in her approach while undertaking treatment. Her speech should be clear and if necessary with particular effort to make contact by facing the patient, or by touch if he cannot see well. If she detects his morale is low she will have to be careful that urging, or even teasing, is not perceived as bullying. (Refusal of treatment was discussed in Chapter 2, pp. 34–5.)

Facilitation of short-term memory recall will be assisted if instructions are kept simple. If the patient has dementia this feature has to be skilfully done. Written or verbal advice may be taken quite readily, but if it is to be remembered should be quite brief. A sensitive approach is required in making contact with the other carers whether at home or in an institution. So much unnecessary anxiety is avoided and possible activity maintained if the carer's opinion and the physiotherapist's advice have been communicated effectively.

Social factors

Current social factors that have a bearing on treatment are those relating to life in an old people's home. In such a public existence the immobile patients may not always be willing to practise an individual exercise with others watching. The level of staffing seldom allows regular help or supervision of activities unless they are incorporated into the daily programme. A convenient time to enable someone who would need assistance to stand for example, might be during the washing and dressing periods when he could be safe holding onto a wash basin and ease the care assistant's task. An exercise for a patient after a fractured neck of humerus could be in wiping down a table after meals. Some patients who live alone may seldom have visitors, so if asked to practise an exercise it should be simple and safe enough when performed alone.

Length of session and frequency of practice

Delay in central processing in the brain which may be caused by changes in physiology or neurochemistry is not unusual. A 20% increase in reaction time has been assessed between adults of 20 and 60 years (Cole, 1985). This is likely to continue into old age. When this is related to treatment it will be realized that enough time must be allowed for new concepts to be learned, decisions to be taken and physical activity to be initiated as well as completed at each session. Despite an extended time scale, there is not necessarily any loss of learning ability.

Since the cardiovascular system is less effective, rests will have to be allowed more frequently than a young fit adult would have thought necessary. Bone healing takes the same length of time for people of all ages but full recovery of muscle strength and joint range may be slower because of the lesser amount of exercise that is possible. Other pathology would be a more important reason for increasing the time scale for a course of treatment and the setbacks that might delay a steady recovery.

Elderly patients in hospital who are frail either physically or mentally would manage the effort of activity or of concentration for only brief episodes. In order to reinforce the effect of treatment, frequent repetition would be more effective.

Compromises due to multipathology

In a survey conducted by Mark Abrams of people at home aged 75 and over only 10% claimed to have no problems (Abrams, 1978). The average person reported 6 of the 21 ailment descriptions, the most common being arthritis, unsteadiness, forgetfulness and poor eyesight. This is not surprising to anyone working with older patients, but the implications for treatment are obvious and the problems sometimes baffling.

The problems can be a combination of the reason for referral, plus a number of previous residual pathologies both reported by the patient and those discovered after examination or added even after treatment has commenced.

Example: Mr Bush may perhaps have begun to make some recovery following a stroke despite partial loss of movement and sensation in his left side. Only when he stands does an osteoarthritic knee begin

76

to give trouble, thus limiting the time he can be on his feet, and preventing kneeling as a balance activity. Knee extension exercises in sitting would be inadvisable for fear of provoking associated reactions so other pain-relieving and knee-stabilizing methods would be adopted.

Splints, callipers or spinal corsets are often provided to support a limb or spine for reasons of pain or weakness. Some may be worn for many years, but in the course of time the shape and girth of limbs may change so that if the support is still required, it and the body part, should be checked. This is true also of lower limb prostheses. The condition of the skin over bony points might need extra protection. Increasing weakness or deformity of hands might cause the task of fastening the straps and buckles to be more difficult or even impossible, and easier methods might have to be devised if the support continues to be essential. Although splints or corsets might be considered useful in pain relief, other conditions sometimes prevent their being worn. Abdominal pressure imposed by wearing a corset would increase the dyspnoea of a chest condition.

The choice of walking aids may be affected by conflicting situations, both pathological and practical. Even if a walking frame is a sound choice to give a patient confidence and control unsteadiness, pain in the back or shoulders might be worsened by having to lift it forward. He might manage better at home without having anything to carry except a stick if furniture were situated to provide support. Although a patient with a hip replacement who manages to walk confidently in a physiotherapy department using sticks, the anxiety caused by crossing the open spaces of a residential home could render this venture impossible so that a walking frame would be preferred to promote independence.

Chest treatment may require modification. Postural drainage as treatment for bronchiectasis might well have to be adapted if the patient also has an osteoarthritic hip or suffers with cardiac failure.

Some patients at any age have multiple problems, but the incidence in old age is more common, and the type more likely to be degenerative which influences the energy level at which activity is continued. Physiotherapy is most severely altered if multipathology includes mental illness. Being sensitive to the patient's reactions, conduct of treatment has to be slow, with obvious purpose and in short sessions. Multipathology while presenting a challenge for ingenuity in adapting treatments, is not a pretext for avoiding the attempt.

Involvement of carers

While most patients, whether at home or in hospital, have family and friends who visit, help and take an interest, with increasing age many of the former tend to rely heavily on this support. For some patients this is provided by home helps, and other social service employees. Some have district nurses, some voluntary scheme visitors. Many of those in hospital depend on nurses for physical assistance or encouragement for moving about if not for all activity. This can be the situation at any age of course but more likely in later years.

One obvious difference is that the family member if spouse or sibling may be equally frail. Physiotherapists could waste much rehabilitation time and cause unnecessary distress if inadequate attention is given to listening to and guiding the carer, thus minimizing effort and reducing anxiety levels.

Anyone who has to care for a sick elderly or disabled loved one is bound to experience a number of psychological difficulties and problems. It is important that the relative is enabled to recognize the problems and realize that they are normal. This is achieved in part by the members of the caring team who listen attentively and acknowledge the worries. There are often feelings of bewilderment on the part of a carer and inadequacy in attempts to deal with the patient's pain and incapacity, especially in the unfamiliar setting of hospital. There can be difficulties for relatives in developing adequate relationships with hospital staff in order to have enough trust to ask questions.

Many carers are taught handling skills with explanation, demonstration and then 'now it's your turn' methods. In the teaching of handling skills to older home carers, the therapist should be alert for signs of their physical discomfort or anxiety. If enquiries elicit report of pain which is aggravated by the suggested method of handling then some adaptation may be required. What seems an easy movement for a young and strong physiotherapist may cause considerable worry to an elderly family member. If the necessary procedure remains too difficult despite alterations, this points to a need for social service or nursing assistance at home. Some elderly carers may not be aware of what help is available or reluctant to ask.

When the initial strains and stresses have been experienced, there may be longer-term difficulties for a family carer that a physiotherapist should appreciate when suggesting co-operation with

78

treatment. These include stress with the accompanying physical symptoms, feelings of depression and loneliness. If the patient has severe mental illness, his carer may well suffer a prolonged bereavement reaction of grief and guilt. Especially in the case of child and parent there may be difficulty in role reversal (Spragg, 1984).

Given the amount of extra labour as well as strain some carers cope with, if the patient is at home but not physically independent, the home carer may consider she has enough to do without a lot of extra tasks involved with the patient's home work.

It may seem to suit her better if he remains fixed in a chair 'so he won't get up and fall on the floor and I can't pick him up'. That point of view should be given attention and the real reason assessed if thought to be an excuse. The inappropriate wandering about is one of the least well-tolerated habits by a home carer, with incontinence, aggression and feeding difficulties (Argyle, Jestice and Brooks, 1985). This may point to a need for referral to a social worker about organizing temporary relief.

In some long-term care institutions a 'key worker' is identified which, for the physiotherapist, simplifies greatly the task of agreeing levels of patient activity or methods of assistance. She has to deal with that one care assistant or nurse only who acts as a friend to the patient and liaison agent with other workers.

Health education in prevention of accident or avoidable deterioration

Although health education tends to form a part of every patient's physiotherapy management, it is probably more broadly based for older patients. Due to the likelihood of degenerative conditions, or normal ageing, informed advice in the appropriate amount is often useful. Sometimes this may be in positive encouragement to do more rather than less, thus demoting false myths of ageism. Educating the patient during treatment of chronic or degenerative disease on how to manage the condition should reduce the perceived need or demand for regular repeat course of 'more physiotherapy'. Repeat requests may be justified when patients have inflammatory episodes of joint disease or when stroke-disabled patients stiffen up following an illness. Each course, however, may need to be no more than re-education and re-encouragement. (See also Chapter 6.)

79

5

Working as a team

Rowena Kinsman

Effective care of patients requires co-operation of all team members. These will include all those concerned with the patients' management and support.

WHAT IS A TEAM?

In society teamwork is seen in a large number of professions and organizations. This may be a consequence of increased scientific knowledge and over-expanding areas of specialization, as well as a change in the way businesses have become corporations and multinational firms. Teamwork refers to a group of people who make different contributions towards the achievement of a common goal.

Teamwork implies a commitment and a purpose. For example, in a football team there are eleven members to a team. Each member knows his place, where he will be playing and what is expected of him. There is an involvement and a commitment to win the game. At the end of the game the team will meet to discuss the game. Individual team members will share their thoughts as to how the game might have gone. If the team is well known, it will have its followers, who will evaluate the game and comment in minute detail. There may be consequences, for example, one player may be dropped from the team and another one brought in. Whatever the changes the team will be committed to improving their performance. No one team member can be too involved in this commitment.

80

WHY IS THERE SUCCESS OR FAILURE?

Physiotherapists are used to working with other physiotherapists and in general have no problem sharing thoughts as to how a patient might be treated in an outpatient department for example. Usually the more experienced physiotherapist takes the lead in setting treatment goals and deciding upon a plan of action. However, when the physiotherapist works on the wards it is not so easy for immediately there are more people to deal with, for instance, the nurse and the doctor. Each person has his/her goals for the patient and so the analogy with the football team is not so clear. Although each member of the health care team is committed the goal for each professional may not be the same. For example, the nurse may be concerned that the patient gets to the toilet not how the patient gets there, which may be the physiotherapist's concern.

In the Health Service, there is a lot of confusion about teamwork. The literature is full of jargon and often there is the assumption that teamwork is cheaper, although there is no evidence to suggest this. In part, this may be a consequence of the way teamwork developed in the Health Service. There used to be a passive acceptance of the routine tasks. These were handed down by the physician and the nurse.

Alongside this, professions have developed and no longer is the Health Service dominated by the medical profession. There are many professions involved in the delivery of health care. They can be employed by either Health or Social Services, or may even be employed by a voluntary organization. A partnership is developed between the different professionals, often referred to as the multi-disciplinary team. In theory each team member unites his/her efforts to provide the best possible care for the patient. In practice there are many problems in establishing an effective health care system. The main problems are tradition, training and communication. Using the analogy of a football team, there is clearly a difference between a football team and a multidisciplinary team. The football team has a captain who decides who will play. In the multidisciplinary team, often there is no identifiable leader. The different professions do not know precisely what each has to offer.

Tradition

At one time it was not uncommon for a doctor to ask for heat and

81

exercises for a painful shoulder. The patient with a painful shoulder believed he/she was coming to physiotherapy for massage. The doctor was not trained as a physiotherapist and was therefore not familiar with treatment regimes. The patient went on hearsay. Neither the doctor requesting a specific treatment nor the patient's beliefs are now thought to be helpful in a multidisciplinary team. Another example would be an inappropriate referral such as an elderly lady attending physiotherapy for difficulty with walking who would do better to go initially to chiropody to have her feet treated and be advised on foot care.

Training

It is difficult for the professions to share knowledge when each health profession has its own training system (Pritchard, 1981). For example, in physiotherapy, students are taught in isolation by their professional peers. During this period there is little opportunity to meet with doctors, nurses and other staff employed to provide health care. It is, therefore, hardly surprising that professionals have difficulty coming to terms with sharing care when qualifying. Post-registration training could possibly tackle many of the problems. However, there are no statutory requirements for the post-registration training of paramedical professions and few for the other allied professions. What training there is, is largely concerned with the teaching of professional skills rather than with joint learning. Professional skills are again taught in isolation and are in no way structured, although some professional associations are attempting to standardize training, and working towards a more professional standard by offering degree courses. It is not easy for each profession to know what the other has to offer, nevertheless it should be possible for each professional to say whether or not they can help a patient achieve a goal. As a consequence of this *ad hoc* training, the professions have developed into areas that traditionally have been the domain of other professions, for example, counselling skills where the development has been in direct response to patient need. The role of each profession is now less easy to define. For example, nurses not only nurse, they assess, treat, advise, rehabilitate and co-ordinate the services going to the patient. Often this latter role is difficult to achieve if other professions do not have a regular commitment and are not consistent in when they see a patient. For example, it is not a good idea if the physiotherapist visits a patient on the same day as the bathing attendant and the chiropodist.

Development of overlapping skills

As with nursing, similar changes can be seen in physiotherapy, where therapists have moved out into the community, seeing patients in their own homes. They may work in psychiatry, care of the dying and industry, to name but a few examples. These changes have, to a large extent, gone on in each profession unrecognized by the others, so that there is now considerable overlap (Figure 5.1) between what the different professions do, thereby making it increasingly difficult to establish shared care.

Figure 5.1 Role of physiotherapy and nursing.

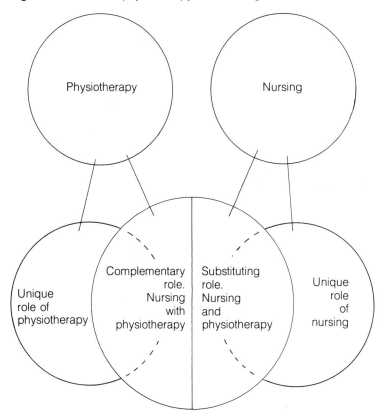

Besides there being an area of overlap there is a need for some professionals to do the work of others, that is substitute when they do not work. For example, physiotherapists normally work a nine-to-five day, only doing emergency duties out of those hours. A unique role for a physiotherapist working with a repaired fractured neck of femur may be to teach the patient to walk again initially using a walking frame. The nurses overlap with the physiotherapists in that they, too, work to rehabilitate the patient to independence and so they would encourage the patient to walk and substitute for the physiotherapist on the weekend, ensuring that the patient does walk. Unfortunately it is often difficult to perform the substituting role satisfactorily owing to staffing pressure, emergencies, unexpected visitors, to name but a few examples. This may lead to frustration as the nurse would be unable to do the nursing role. There is no satisfactory solution; however, if each profession understands the other's role it does help.

Each profession is managed by a member of its own profession. Physiotherapists are managed by district physiotherapists or superintendent physiotherapists. There is a professional hierarchy. The district physiotherapist sets objectives and monitors physiotherapy care, while observing professional autonomy as laid down by the professional association. For a relatively new and largely unproven profession such as physiotherapy, there is an observed need to defend one's roles, which sometimes makes it difficult to share in teamwork. For example, at a team meeting a physiotherapist may say a patient can walk with minimal assistance, however, the nurses may experience difficulties. Unless the physiotherapist shares her knowledge it is not possible for the nurses to walk the patient with minimal assistance.

Status and leadership

Physiotherapists, unlike nurses, receive their training in college and are supernumerary to the department staffing when they do their clinical practice. Student nurses, on the other hand, are a critical part of the work force. The entry requirements for a student nurse in general are lower than those for entering physiotherapy training, implying that a qualified physiotherapist has a higher status in the eyes of the public than a nurse. This can be taken further with the medical student, who has an even higher entry requirement than a physiotherapist and needs five years at university. Although this may

84

mean that the doctor is the most knowledgeable person in the team, does it necessarily mean that he/she should be the leader of the team that provides the best possible care to the patient? There is a wide variety of opinion regarding leadership of teamwork. In the analogy with the football team, one player is chosen to be the captain. He is chosen for his leadership qualities and through proven experience. Some doctors believe that leadership should be shared. Still others suggest that the person taking the initiative at any one time should be the leader and that this can rotate. Leadership is a complex issue and needs to be dealt with if teamwork is to work in practice. There is little opportunity to train, either by example or by attending courses. Apart from the doctors the turnover of staff in the other professions is high so that the team members are always changing. An understanding of the different professional roles can help lesson the effect of staff change over.

Communication

A team should be no bigger than is needed to provide the best possible standard of care. Deciding the size of a team is sometimes difficult and it may be helpful to examine who is with the patient most of the day, after the normal working day and during the weekend. This often tends to be a relative or a nurse if the patient is in hospital. Whoever it is needs to know what he/she should do in order to provide the best standard of care and in the case of rehabilitation the opportunities for the patient to practise what he/she needs to learn, so as to function to maximum potential. Each member of a team should be able to take part in the team's activities and feel free to express ideas that are relevant to patient care. Communication in any team is difficult and often breaks down with each profession resorting to its own professional jargon. Although there is a move to get away from professional terminology, there is a need to have a team language, a language that is shared. This is acquired by each member of the team sharing his/her basic concepts and philosophy. A sympathetic attitude to each other's objectives and methods of functioning is then established. This is done by careful planning and discussion. There is a need to meet regularly. A common failure of the multidisciplinary team is the lack of regular meetings. Often meetings take place once a week, or fortnight which makes it almost impossible for each team member to contribute towards creating realistic goals. For example, if on initial assessment, the physiotherapist decides the goal for a patient should

85

be independent chair transfers, this goal might not be achieved by the first team meeting, one week later. The reason for this could be that the patient was seen by many different professionals each of whom practised a slightly different method of transfer. The patient can easily be confused by different instructions and end up by taking the easiest way out. Some times this is not the best method.

On the hand, if each person involved with the patient had agreed on independent chair transfers initially, both the goal and the achievement of it would have been shared. This would have contributed to a consistent approach, simplifying the situation for the patient and providing an earlier opportunity for success.

The lengths of team meetings may vary depending upon the needs of its different members. The meetings are facilitated by a neutral venue. All too often professionals have their own department headquarters in which to retreat and there is no suitable place for a mixed group to meet. They resort to meeting on a ward, in a secretary's office, or somewhere also equally unsuitable.

It is important that when a meeting takes place there is adequate seating for all those attending. It is helpful to have an agenda so that everyone comes prepared and to have also an agreed time for the meeting.

For communication to be complete, it is important that records of meetings and of patient care are kept. The latter should be shared, so that each member is aware of change. Problem-orientated medical records are one system of record keeping that has evolved and incorporates a record common to all members of the team, regardless of the need to keep more detailed individual records. Whatever system of record keeping is chosen, it is important that each member of the team has access to the notes (see pp. 131, 134).

WHAT ARE THE PATTERNS OF RELATIONSHIPS?

Various descriptions and definitions of team work have been described and there is broad agreement that in primary health care work there is a model (Figure 5.2) that accommodates most of the variations. This model always allows for the general practitioner, nurse and patient (Pritchard, 1984). These three roles may be described as the nucleus of a team. The doctor and the nurse share knowledge. Sometimes there is a need to ask other services to intervene or advise on a consultancy basis, or to provide support services (Figure 5.3).

Figure 5.2 Pattern of relationships in the basic model of a primary health care team.

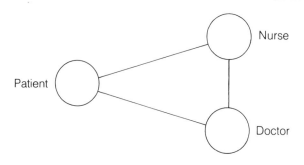

Figure 5.3 Model of primary health care team including support services, in this case consultancy.

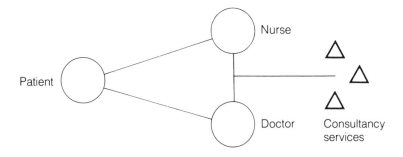

Consultancy services could be home helps, meals on wheels, or bathing attendants to name a few. When other services are employed it is important that they are co-ordinated, for example, when arranging the home help it may be helpful to the patient if the day did not clash with the district nurse visit. This may take the form of a telephone conversation, letter and/or telephone call.

On occasion it is necessary to seek the help of other professionals, for example, physiotherapists, chiropodists (Figure 5.4). Usually the general practitioner contacts the physiotherapist who assesses the patient and decides whether to treat and/or give advice.

A patient with Parkinson's disease may be referred for physiotherapy and the therapist decides that the patient does not need a course of treatment but that the relatives need advice in handling. Occasionally the physiotherapist may need to turn to a professional

87

Figure 5.4 Model of primary health care team including other professionals, in this case physiotherapists.

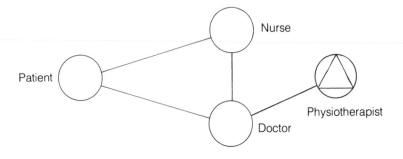

Figure 5.5 Model of primary health care team, including the physiotherapist, where a senior physiotherapist is called for further advice.

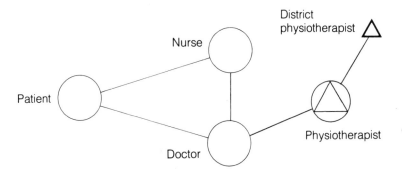

superior for further advice (Figure 5.5). For example, the patient referred may have had a recent stroke, on top of there being an above-knee amputation on the unaffected side. The district physiotherapist would through experience be able to advise.

Sometimes many professionals are involved in the case of a patient and for purposes of consistency it is decided to have a key worker for one or more patients. For example, on a long-stay ward a nurse may be the keyworker. A physiotherapist may show the nurse how to facilitate a patient to roll over and get out of bed so that the patient actively does the movement. Another example would be an

Table 5.1 Members of a team

Non health care professionals	Health care professionals
receptionist	doctor
home help	nurse
helper	occupational therapist
relative	physiotherapist
domestic helper	dietitian
friend	speech therapist
milkman	social worker
grocer	psychologist
hairdresser	
secretary	
administrator	
priest	
volunteer	
teacher	

untrained person who is employed and trained by professionals to help a person function to maximum potential.

In the community a relative is often the main carer. In the case of the elderly it is especially important that all those professionals involved teach the relative how best to handle the patient. The relative may be elderly, have health problems or difficulty in moving easily. If the relative is to cope he/she needs to be shown what to do, know what to expect and be confident that when he/she needs help it will be forthcoming. Professional staff need to recognize who is doing the caring, listen to the carer's reports and observations before making decisions to change the patient's management. When defining teams it is important to include all those who come into contact with the patient's episode of care. Many of these persons may not be directly involved with the patient but their work is vital to the functioning of the nuclear team. For example, in a general practitioner's office, the first person a patient speaks to is the receptionist. It is, therefore, important that the receptionist knows how to help a patient with advice about who best to see and make the necessary arrangements. More often that not, the patient's first contact with the health service is the receptionist who, by showing concern, starts off the episode of health care effectively. The receptionist, together with others, may be included at any one time with a large number of different agencies who need to be co-ordinated (Table 5.1).

It is easy for the nuclear team, especially in primary health care, to meet regularly and review the patient case load, working arrangements, communication and any other topics of mutual interest. The patient and the carer would not be present at such meetings as many cases will be discussed. In the hospital such meetings take place among the doctors and nurses on wards but immediately other professionals are involved they become large and unwieldy. The doctor and the nurse are primarily concerned with nursing and medical functions. When the professionals are called in, other aspects of care come into play, for example, rehabilitation may be covered by physiotherapists, occupational therapists and social workers. These professionals need to be co-ordinated and develop paths of communication, so that everyone shares the patient's goals. Meetings should be organized on a regular basis. They should be short and to the point and only for those persons involved in the care of the patient. Occasionally there is a need to involve everyone in a meeting. The purpose of large meetings should be clear, for example in a general practice surgery it is useful to have all persons working in the practice get together. Such meetings should have an agenda and need to include educational topics as well as opportunities for staff to learn about each others' skills. The agenda should be of interest to all those attending if it is not to break up into little private conversations.

Besides team meetings it is important that each profession examines its own professional skills. To do this it is necessary for individual professions to have meetings on their own. These meetings should be structured so that junior staff are able to learn and also be supported in their role. For example nurses in one group practice may meet to discuss the management of incontinence. They may also bring in a consultant to advise them on latest theory and practice, or attend courses on a local or national level. Sometimes one or two professions can combine in their training needs, for example, nurses and physiotherapists in the factured neck of femur. Nurses need to know how a patient can move and physiotherapists depend upon the nurse input in order for the patient to practise and improve his/her mobility.

HOW IS IT DIFFERENT WITH OLDER PATIENTS?

When working with elderly patients who have a complexity of problems and are needing an input from many professions, it is necessary for each professional to know what their own contribution

90

brings in terms of special gerontological knowledge and how to support the contributions of others. This knowledge is acquired from many sources one of the most important being experience – including observation, listening and discussion. Practice in each profession not only has individual character and local variations, but it changes generally over time. Knowledge of much of this will not be available in written form but must be sought locally.

Thus forearmed it is possible to identify all those people who may be involved with the patient's episode of care and to choose a small nuclear team. This team then identifies the goals that the team is working toward. In rehabilitation these goals should be shared with the patient and can be broken down into long-term, intermediate and short-term goals (see Chapter 3).

In order to achieve the goals the nuclear team needs to consult with other professions and then decide together how best the plans should be implemented.

In sharing the care of elderly people in a consistent and humane manner, a feature that relates to the team's effectiveness can be attitudes to being old or helpless, to long-term care, or death. This may require discussion in the group, otherwise misunderstandings could affect joint planning.

All this understanding can take years to achieve but an adverse factor is often the frequent changes of staff in geriatric units. Physiotherapy with older patients does not always arouse interest or enjoy high status despite the demanding nature of the work. One survey found that only 9% of 100 physiotherapists were prepared to work in geriatric care on a long-term basis (Finn, 1986). Attitudes to older people, however, were on the whole positive. Physiotherapy students' response to working on geriatric units was markedly influenced by others (Squires and Simpson, 1987). Thus, team members may need to make positive efforts to support each other, especially when there are dispiriting influences.

With collaboration and mutual understanding, the care given by the team can be greater than the sum of individual care. Specialist skills are used well and as a result there is increased job satisfaction.

6

Maintenance of good health

Patricia Smith

An efficient physiotherapy service includes the provision of advice on prevention of unnecessary problems and encouraging the patient to achieve optimum levels of independence and health.

WHAT IS GOOD HEALTH?

Maintenance of good health means staying healthy, prevention of disability or chronic ill-health in elderly people. Diet and exercise play an important part in this and it is in the latter area of exercise and general advice, in terms of prevention of problems, where the physiotherapist has a prime role. Many elderly people are under the misapprehension that exercise is something that children and young adults do compulsively, the middle-aged foolishly and the elderly not at all. However, it can be seen that if older people become less active the muscles provide less stimulation and therefore the body becomes out of condition. This leads to increasing weakness and loss of function and mobility of the individual which many come to associate with growing older but this is not always directly attributable to advancing years. This increasing inactivity leads to tiredness and lethargy which is not relieved by rest. Only exertion can produce the type of sleep necessary to replenish the body's biochemical balance thus producing extra potential energy for the body to use to perpetuate vitality or a zest for life.

To promote good health some elderly people need to expand their range of physical and mental activity, and exercise has a beneficial effect on all the body's systems helping to maintain the best possible function.

WHEN DOES MAINTENANCE BEGIN?

When considering the subject of maintenance of good health, we may ask the question, when does good health begin? Good health usually begins before birth and lays the foundation for health in old age. By and large the population is now able to achieve a higher standard of health, thanks to primary prevention of disease such as better standards of living with improved sanitation and more advanced health care. For example with preconceptual and genetic advice and better antenatal care, the incidence of certain hereditary problems and conditions has been considerably reduced, e.g. Down's syndrome and spina bifida. Also improved medical treatment has enabled some persons to expect a longer life, for example the Parkinson's disease sufferer. There are, however, factors to be considered during our stages of life to maintain good health and one of the most important is the development of good habits, such as diet, exercise, early treatment of ailments, non-abuse of alcohol and drugs. These habits cannot begin too early if an individual is to have the best possible chance of a long and healthy life. The physiotherapist has a definite role to play in this health education, particularly in the area of secondary prevention. This involves teaching people how to prevent unnecessary deformities, muscle wasting or joint stiffness, general care of joints to avoid further damage in osteoarthritis and reducing or avoiding the risk of repetition of certain conditions such as back and shoulder injuries. An educative role in primary prevention may take place in schools dealing with subjects such as back care and exercise.

Much of the physiotherapist's work in this area is centred around the principle of 'Prevention is better than cure'. Many elderly people need advice on how to maintain good health and how to foster a positive attitude to the expectation of growing old. Health at any age gives the individual the advantage of choice in life. Many people, as they grow older, come to expect an inevitable loss of this element of choice due to the misapprehension that increasing age and increasing physical and mental infirmity go hand in hand. Therefore, there is a general negative attitude to ageing, which in turn creates an ageing population with little will or enthusiasm to maintain or improve their healthy status. People make adaptations to their life style as they age to make things easier for themselves. Such things as swapping their house for a bungalow to eliminate the effort of climbing stairs or sitting down to put socks or tights on, thus avoiding standing on one leg. Although these adaptations may be necessary if health problems have arisen, older generally fit people do themselves no favours by less use of their physical capabilities. The old saying 'What you don't use, you lose' applies firmly to this group and here is another area in which the physiotherapist can educate elderly people in the best ways to maintain their life style and make full use of physical resources. The correct advice and support can enable them to adapt both mentally and physically to any necessary changes in their life brought about by certain conditions which may affect them as they grow older, for example osteoarthritis and hemiplegia. Good health is not age related but is relevant to each individual and many people can live successfully independent lives despite having experienced illnesses. Feeling well is normal regardless of age and the elderly person should be encouraged to seek help from the doctor if they feel consistently tired, listless or generally unwell as this is often a sign of pathological illness and not to be accepted under the umbrella of 'What else can I expect? I'm not getting any younger'. To be able to appreciate the difference between feeling ill and being healthy a change in thinking is needed to create a positive attitude to health in old age. This change in thinking is needed early on in life to reverse the general trend of the next generation's attitude to their ability to be healthy in later life. There is now an increasing awareness in the younger generation of how diet and regular exercise can lead to a healthier life style in later years. The media, in the form of television, radio and newspapers, has a large part to play in continuing this change of attitude and thinking. The plight of the sick elderly is thrust upon us from every visible angle to highlight deficiencies in National Health Service care, which does nothing to inform us of the advantages of life for the predominantly healthy older population. Few, if any, articles or programmes appear to educate people in promoting health and fitness in retirement or to provide information about agencies and organizations that can help in this field. Despite the media's insistence on dealing with the ailing elderly, if we look around us we are surrounded by ever-increasing numbers of fit retired people in our shopping areas, on coach tours, or on package holidays abroad, all enjoying their healthy later years and the freedom of choice to do as they please with them.

Hereditary factors play a part in good health in later years. There are families who can be considered a biological elite who live to advanced ages, sharing very few, if any, of the signs and symptoms we have long associated with great age. These people often achieve great things in their 80s and 90s and are always ready to meet challenges both physical and mental. Heredity we can do nothing about but control of our environment and life style we can. To maintain good health the elderly person, if a smoker should give up, improve his diet and take some gentle regular exercise, thereby reversing some of his negative environment or offsetting a weaker constitution dealt to him by his family history. This highlights a need for education in such matters which the physiotherapist is more than able to provide.

WHO CAN HELP?

The physiotherapist plays a major role in the maintenance of health in the elderly population but she is only one of a vast number of agencies available to give help and support where needed. The physiotherapist needs to be aware of all these other agencies to foster the vital link between the elderly patients in her care and these agencies as well as using these resources to increase her own experience in order to advise others. The most useful of these agencies are:

The media

Television, radio, magazines and newspapers are the most widespread resources keeping elderly people in touch with the outside world. The media play a dual role both in conveying improvements and advice to elderly people such as news of new research findings and also in educating all age groups on matters concerning the health and welfare of our senior citizens. Less mobile elderly people rely heavily on the media for information and there are more and more television and radio programmes and written articles on health matters and points of interest for this group but still by no means sufficient in relation to this large and ever-increasing group.

Voluntary disease-related organizations

Over the years many groups have been set up to bring together people who are suffering from the effects of various diseases and several of these organizations can be of direct help to elderly people. These groups such as the Parkinson Disease Society and the Chest, Heart and Stroke Association, can give great support to both sufferers of

95

disease and their carers. This support can take the form of general information about the disease, its causes and effects and current research and treatment, or direct links with other sufferers or carers via local support groups where experiences can be shared, which helps to relieve the isolation and desolation of coping with increasing disability through disease. Some associations such as the Parkinson's Disease Society or Multiple Sclerosis Society also arrange holidays for patients where treatment is available and the effects of a change of scenery and some intensive physiotherapy can have very beneficial effects for elderly people suffering from these diseases. Age Concern is one of the voluntary organizations most directly concerned with the welfare of the elderly population, running frequent campaigns and producing a great deal of literature on all aspects of coping with life after retirement.

Mutual support schemes

There is no greater motivated group in the quest for a healthy old age than elderly people themselves. All over the country various mutual support schemes are being set up to bring these people together for fellowship and support. These schemes may take the form of luncheon clubs, pensioners' clubs or women's organizations such as the Women's Institute and many of these clubs are run by the fit elderly themselves.

At these clubs elderly people can meet for social events as well as have an opportunity to listen to regular speakers talking on health issues and other topics related to the elderly population and its survival. Carers can also benefit greatly from the support of others involved in similar situations, as caring for an elderly disabled person can be both demanding and isolating. The Association of Carers provides a network of support groups and information on a range of subjects connected with the care of handicapped and elderly people. In some areas an idea from the United States of America has been adopted and retired people are being trained as counsellors under a 'Peer Health Counselling' scheme enabling the elderly to advise their own generation on health maintenance, thus relieving some of the pressure on the medical agencies. The people involved in this scheme have found it easier to talk to their counsellor who is 'one of us' and therefore understands certain feelings and problems and communication is easier than with the doctor from the point of view of time available and language. Another scheme being tried out is the 'Senior Health Shop', where older people can drop in for coffee or a snack and have their blood pressure checked by a qualified nurse, and answer a computerized questionnaire on health as well as gathering any information on health care they may need. Other ideas along these lines are being tried out; there is a great movement in this direction of self help and various existing organizations are being asked to help, the University of the Third Age being particularly involved.

Aids advisory services

Rehabilitation engineering movement advisory panel

This is a network of professional volunteers comprising engineers, technicians, chemists etc., who come together specifically to solve certain problems of individual disabled persons. They will produce 'one off' aids and adaptations to existing aids very promptly enabling elderly people to live independently or to improve the quality of their existing care.

Disabled living foundation

Aids for elderly or handicapped persons are continually changing and improving and many different manufacturers are involved in the production of aids for the disabled. Most countries have aids centres such as the Disabled Living Foundation in Great Britain, which are regional centres where all aids for the disabled are on display and can be tried out by any one who may be interested. Examples of these aids vary widely from adapted baths and shower cubicles to small items like tap turners and adapted plugs. The Disabled Living Foundation is staffed by a variety of different personnel including occupational therapists and physiotherapists, as well as disabled members of staff who will test various aids and are, therefore, able to give first-hand information to clients. The staff of the Disabled Living Foundation are in direct contact with the manufacturers who are constantly updating aids and producing new ones and some manufacturers will produce 'one off' aids for specific clients if requested. The services of the Foundation are available for any elderly person or their carers for personal visits to see what aids are available. They produce a regular catalogue of aids and information sheets on various subjects which are of great assistance to the physiotherapist working with the elderly.

97

Social services

Every local authority has a Social Services Department. These vary considerably from district to district in terms of the resources they can offer to elderly people to enable them to maintain good health. These resources may take the form of provision of day centres staffed by social workers and volunteers and the supply of walking and other aids to elderly people to enable them to live independently. If necessary the social services department may provide home improvements or adaptations, for example building a downstairs shower room or toilet or installing a stair-lift. These arrangements will be made by an occupational therapist. Social workers or their assistants may advise on financial matters such as claims for supplementary benefit or attendance allowance or arrange home help, or respite care for families caring for disabled people. Social services may also provide a meals on wheels service which can be a vital source of nutrition of an elderly person as well as providing a social contact. The latter is a bonus and is not a reason for a service. It is important that the need for any service is carefully assessed.

Churches

Many churches run pensioners' clubs, luncheon clubs or day centres, where members of their congregation and local residents can get together to give each other mutual support and friendship. By virtue of their humanitarian feelings, all religious groups are in a position to help elderly people to maintain their health by providing transport to get them out of their homes and more involved in the community, thus removing from them the feeling of isolation which is such a destructive factor in later life. Youth organizations attached to churches, synagogues etc. do a lot of voluntary work for old people, such as gardening, decorating etc., which prevents the elderly from taking unnecessary risks tackling jobs which they may not be able to manage. Many people in later life also derive a great deal of spiritual and emotional help from their religious beliefs and their ability to be part of a religious community. This helps their morale and their mental approach towards ageing, and acts as a positive factor in the maintenance of good health.

Carers at home

Carers can be used to describe anyone that cares for another – be they families, friends, volunteers or health-care professionals, each one has a lot to offer the older person in terms of advice and practical help. Carers must understand the need for the elderly to remain independent and their pride in this and only help when it is absolutely necessary – perhaps having given the elderly person the opportunity to try something unaided themselves at first, only stepping in to help when they are in difficulties. The carer must always guard against being over protective, thus taking away the elderly person's autonomy and also respect the person's desire to tackle a task in their own way. 'Old habits die hard' is a saying to be taken into consideration when caring for or helping elderly people. Many older people can be persuaded to change some of their habits for the better, if given a sound reason but sometimes 'old dogs can't learn new tricks'. One should always be prepared for helpful advice to be ignored, habit and resistance to change is inherent in the older generation and carers should not be put off from continuing to offer help and support after some initial rejection. The physiotherapist, whilst playing a caring role for the patient, must also fulfill her role of caring for the carers. This will involve teaching correct handling and lifting techniques in order to maintain the health of the carer.

Residential home care staff

Helping the elderly people in residential homes to keep healthy is a vital role of the care staff. Many people entering residential homes will have some problems in mobility and self care and it is very important that they be encouraged to maintain their independence for as long as possible. This is both essential for the resident's morale and attitude to life and the more dependent on the staff the residents become, the more this will become a problem. Organizing social events, activity groups and exercise sessions will help to keep these people healthy. Many old people's homes, both private and local authority funded, have regular visits from physiotherapists to advise the staff on the management of the residents' physical problems and the best way to maintain or improve their levels of functional independence. They also teach the staff correct lifting and handling of the residents to prevent injury to the care staff, many of whom are unqualified.

WHAT NEEDS SEEING TO?

Having considered these other agencies who are able to help both the elderly and the physiotherapist involved in their care, it is now necessary to consider what factors have a direct effect on the life of these people that may necessitate change to promote good health in later life. If we are to assist in helping elderly people maintain good health, attention to their environment is a must.

Environmental hazards

Many elderly people live in older properties in accommodation which may have been in existence since their youth. As the years pass they are neither aware of the inadequacy of this accommodation and the changes in their specific needs as they age, i.e. the need for two stair rails, more heating etc., nor have they the financial resources to deal with these changes. The physiotherapist has an important role to play in recognizing potential hazards around the home and suggesting modifications and alterations where necessary. This, of course, is only possible where the elderly person concerned is willing to accept the necessary changes. In circumstances where they are living with other family members or friends or they are in rented accommodation, the family, friends or landlord must also be in agreement. Some elderly people are resistant to change and so the physiotherapist must always be prepared for advice given to be politely declined, or ignored altogether on occasions.

The following may be a useful check list when looking for environmental hazards.

1. Access to buildings – steps, lift, stairs, doorway, paths, lighting.
2. Floor coverings – worn and loose carpets, slip mats, lino, worn floorboards, uneven surfaces.
3. Corridors and passageways – poor lighting, narrow access, obstruction by furniture, steps.
4. Furniture – position of items, space around items, general state of repair, height of beds and chairs.
5. Bathrooms – position and height of toilet, access to toilet and bath.
6. Trailing electric flexes.

When looking for hazards the carer must think of the client/patient and decide if there is a hazard, for example loose carpets may cause an elderly person who is unsteady on her feet to trip.

Changes in many of these areas may need the special skills of an occupational therapist but the physiotherapist must be able to advise on these needs to provide safety of movement and the best utilization of the person's physical resources within their own home. Advice may concern such things as not storing heavy items on high shelves to avoid climbing or stretching. Tackling environmental hazards also means checking and advising the individual in the outside environment. The following areas need attention.

1. Walking outdoors – pavements, kerbs, steps, slopes, uneven ground.
2. Transport – getting in and out of cars, on and off buses and trains etc.

This helps the individual to anticipate potential hazards and have the confidence to overcome them.

Physical fitness

One of the many ways in which the physiotherapist can be involved in the maintenance of good health is in giving advice about exercise. Regular exercise helps to maintain the cardiovascular and musculoskeletal systems as well as helping to reduce fatigue and stimulate mental activity. Many elderly people need expert advice on how to modify existing sports that might be taken up at this time of life. As people age and are less able to take part in active sports, the physiotherapist's advice may be valuable in terms of day to day activities. The following areas may need attention.

Posture

This is the basis from which all movement stems and it is therefore very important that good posture should be encouraged and maintained. Postural exercises may need to be taught to enable elderly people to become aware of their posture and how it can be improved. Posture, at rest, is also important if strain on muscles and joints is to be avoided. This can be aided by good use of support, especially chairs and beds.

101

Balance

Poor balance is one of the major contributory factors to falls in the elderly population. Falling leads to loss of confidence and subsequent loss of independence which is to be avoided at all costs. Balance control deteriorates naturally with age and so it is sensible in terms of the maintenance of health to be aware of the mechanisms involved in balance to prevent its loss. Loss of balance occurs when the centre of gravity is displaced and the body cannot accommodate, for example, reaching up to change a light bulb. With a little forethought and the correct advice on base of support, weight transference and head position, accidents can be avoided. However, the best advice would be to avoid these situations that involve reaching upwards, when at all possible. Exercise designed to promote balance should progress from weight transference in sitting and standing and walking to maintenance of balance whilst moving the arms. Walking round obstacles, stepping over things, turning, standing on one leg, stepping on and off a step or stool all help to promote good balance, and teach people how to cope with their altered balance reactions. Elderly people should always be advised to perform balance exercises within reach of something to hold on to, i.e. back of chair, sofa or table.

Lifting

Many people are very active in their retirement years pursuing such hobbies as gardening and do-it-yourself. Inevitably pastimes such as these will involve lifting. For example when gardening one has to turn the soil over, lift potted plants and in general use one's body to achieve a desired result. As long as older people do not have any specific pathology that contra-indicates this activity there is no reason why they should not participate in lifting, as long as correctly instructed in technique. They should be taught the basic rules of:

1. planning the lift
2. widening the base by moving the feet apart
3. bending knees and hips and keeping back straight
4. holding object close to body

However, the best advice on lifting for this group is to lift only when absolutely necessary and then only objects which they can manage easily.

Stairs

Stairs are an excellent source of regular exercise, helping to maintain the quadriceps muscles and the balance mechanisms. They can be safely tackled by all ages and climbing the stairs several times a day will help maintain muscle power and endurance as in any other form of exercise.

General exercise

Many people need specialist advice on the amount of and type of exercise they should maintain in later years. The following factors need to be taken into account:

1. exercises should not cause pain, breathlessness or fatigue
2. endurance needs to be built up slowly either by increasing the number of repetitions or by making the exercise harder, such as by adding weights or lengthening the leverage needed
3. exercises should be done slowly and rhythmically
4. exercises should be done regularly
5. if the person becomes tired or breathless, they should stop the exercise session at that point

Walking

Walking is one of the best forms of exercise for keeping fit and healthy in later life. It has the benefits of being sociable and cheap, does not require any special skills or equipment and it is an outside activity in fresh air. For maximum benefit walking should be fast enough to get out of breath and cover a distance of two miles, three times a week. Joining a ramblers' group may be a good source of fitness and social contact for the more mobile elderly person.

Breathing

In order to remain fit and active, it is necessary to have a good vital capacity in the lungs with efficient gaseous exchange. This prevents fatigue in the muscles and aids mental activity. Vital capacity diminishes with age and may also be affected by smoking or atmospheric pollution, so any exercise programme undertaken by older people should include some breathing exercises to promote lung expansion.

Diet

Maintenance of a good healthy diet should be encouraged by the physiotherapist. Although this is specifically the role of the dietitian, the physiotherapist should be aware of the importance of good diet and by discussion with the elderly person be able to decide whether they need the specialist help of a dietitian or the dental department if feeding or diet seem to be a problem. A well-balanced diet is essential when taking regular exercise. Obesity can reduce mobility and can lead to various pathological conditions such as heart and lung disease, osteoarthritis and diabetes.

Care of the feet

If elderly people are to remain active and healthy it is essential that they have healthy feet. Any activity requiring movement is made extremely difficult if it is performed on painful feet. Advice may be needed on the necessity of keeping toe nails short to avoid pressure on shoes and the easiest positions for reaching the toes to facilitate cutting of the nails. Treatment by a chiropodist may be necessary if there are any specific foot problems or disorders. Many elderly people spend the majority of their time wearing slippers which may not adequately support the feet and if ill-fitting may be a potential cause of falling. Unsuitable footwear can often be a source of painful feet and the importance of correctly supporting footwear must be stressed by the physiotherapist. In certain situations the cushioning effect of trainers may be of value to painful joints in the feet. Examination of the shoes can give the physiotherapist an indication of specific problems with the feet or may lead to investigation of the gait pattern which may have altered, causing soreness of the feet. Equally a foot problem may have altered the gait and these gait and foot disorders need close examination and correct advice on management.

Aids and appliances

Another area in which the elderly person may need the help and advice of a physiotherapist is in the correct choice of aids and appliances, in order to get maximal use from their physical resources. In its simplest form this advice may centre round the best chair for sitting in, with reference to maintenance of good posture and balance involved in getting out of the chair. This may extend to assessment of the need for chair raising blocks or raised toilet seats. Although in many areas these aids may be supplied by an occupational therapist, the physiotherapist must have thorough knowledge of all aids available, and know when it is appropriate to refer for their supply in relation to an elderly person's needs. For example a chair may be simply raised by the patient with the addition of a folded blanket or small pile of newspapers to the seat. The provision of the correct aid or appliance may be all that the person needs to continue to maintain a healthy independent life. The following aids and appliances are those commonly needed by this elderly group:

1. walking aids – sticks, crutches, frames
2. toilet aids – raised seats, rails
3. chair and bed aids – raisers, bed boards, seat raising items
4. wheelchairs
5. splints and callipers
6. corsets and collars
7. surgical shoes and insoles

In this area the physiotherapist's role may also include the making and fitting of certain splints such as collars and insoles, working and resting splints as well as the fitting of 'off the peg' splints and referring the elderly person to an appliance department for others. Advice may also be necessary on correct use of splints or appliances and how the user may wean themselves from them when appropriate.

Social opportunities

Let us now look at social opportunity and its effect on the maintenance of good health in the elderly population. If an elderly person is to remain healthy, he must be able to feel that he is part of a local community, contributing or being involved in it as far as possible. Isolation can be one of the curses of old age and can breed both mental and physical disability as it progresses, although it must be recognized that certain individuals thrive on isolation. One of the greatest barriers for the elderly being involved in community life is transport. Only the more agile members of the ageing population can hop on a bus or train, the less mobile elderly relying heavily on family or friends to transport them in cars whenever possible. With increasing change in the social structure of the family, elderly persons often live far from their families and the majority of their friends are of a similar age which makes getting out and about more of a problem. Some elderly people prefer not to accept too many favours and are therefore grateful for any schemes for car transport where they can pay for a volunteer's petrol or make some contribution.

Having secured transport to their destination, another obstacle to be overcome is access to buildings. Fortunately, as more attention is being drawn to the disabled members of the community, access for wheelchairs, i.e. ramps, make access easier for those elderly people walking thus removing the necessity of using outside steps. Provision of hand rails and lifts in buildings can make a great difference to the elderly population's independence in the community. Certain places where the problem of access needs to be especially considered are:

1. library
2. clinics
3. doctors
4. dentists
5. chiropodists

Example: Miss Brown, a lady of 87, living alone, has recently suffered a Potts fracture after falling down the front steps from her house. Since falling and being put in plaster she has not ventured out and has lost confidence in her ability to walk out of doors unaided. As a result of this time in plaster she is now well overdue for her regular visit to the chiropodist but feels she is unable to negotiate the flight of stone steps up to the chiropodist's house. She cannot take the risk of missing her visit as she suffers from defective circulation to both lower legs and her toe nails need attention but she now feels she must find an alternative chiropodist for the future. As she has no family to call on for help, she has the added worry of finding another chiropodist and as she is at present housebound and reliant on minicabs for transport, this is not an easy task.

Local adult education classes and courses at the University of the Third Age offer a wealth of social opportunity for older people to broaden their horizons and meet new people in the community. The housebound are also able to take courses via the Open University or, in London, can participate in discussions by telephone, which is a recent development by the University of the Third Age. The Health Education Council is very involved in promoting good health in later life, by organizing campaigns to encourage the participation of older people and adult education establishments are often actively involved in these campaigns. All these opportunities, if taken up, can lead to a greatly enhanced quality of life with advancing age and help to keep the mind lively and stimulated, which in turn has beneficial physical effects.

HOW IS IT DIFFERENT WITH OLDER PEOPLE?

Maintenance of good health is an ongoing experience from birth to the end of life. The continuation of this into later life should be no different but sadly, through conditioning and expectation its possibility is ignored.

With reference to the issues mentioned in a previous section of this chapter 'What needs seeing to?', extra difficulties may be presented to some older people. A small number move into convenient accommodation late in life. Most prefer and do remain in the same place for several decades, even over a complete life span, and often without much in the way of change. Old buildings are not necessarily unhealthy but can be damp, cold or dark, the stairs or steps sometimes presenting a risk of stumbling.

One difference that may arise with some older people is that, being accustomed to the dwelling, they may resist any change. The organizing of alterations to a building or the adding of labour-saving devices may be more difficult for very elderly people to organize even if the property is owned and the money is available. Many younger people keep up with material developments by visiting the 'market place' and often have more access to knowledgeable tradesmen.

Lower expectations of health in many older people is based on previous experiences, particularly for those who had little access to medical advice before the advent of the National Health Service. Poor women especially, expected to work hard and to ignore 'minor' complaints. Such individuals in later life are less likely to seek advice, although it may be received gladly enough – if too late for it to be fully effective. Advice may have to take account of fluctuating health and stamina. A partner or carer often bears the strain of encouraging a less fit person to be active and sometimes accepting the risk of accident.

A physiotherapist communicating advice on maintenance of good health may need to ascertain individual or group attitudes to ageing and health before making any assumptions. Although there may be scope for encouraging the captive audience in a club or residential home, much of the information could be passed on via younger friends and relatives. This group, particularly those recently retired, may be the most helpful, enthusiastic and available.

Old age does not have to mean increased disability, and good habits developed during earlier years and continued throughout life can have a dramatic effect on the quality of life in retirement. With increasing numbers of the population now living well over 70 the time has come to challenge unrealistic pessimism and the physiotherapist has a unique role to play in this re-education process and has a duty to promote this in all her dealings with patients of any age, in order to help people achieve a fulfilling and healthy old age.

7

Evaluation and quality assurance

Helen Ransome

Good practice demands that treatments and patterns of management are evaluated in order to check whether the previous six key points have been effective. In order to achieve and maintain optimum standards of service provision, quality assurance programmes should be continuous.

WHAT ARE THEY?

Definitions and tools

Traditionally, along with other health care professionals, physiotherapists have used such phrases as: 'the patient is *much better*'; 'we gave *good treatment* to that patient'; 'we must maintain *high standards* of clinical practice'.

Although each physiotherapist concerned would be quite sure what was meant by these statements, they are subjective. They have no objective meaning, cannot be proved or disproved and certainly cannot be measured. Having recognized this as a problem, an increasing number of brave pioneering physiotherapists set out during the last few decades scientifically to evaluate their clinical practice, discovering in the process why it is easier to be subjective; research and audit in health care are notoriously difficult.

During this period concern was growing in the developed world, including Britain, that the limitation of public spending on health care would lead to arbitrary service cuts and increasingly second-rate services, unless ways could be found of assessing and safeguarding standards of care. At a more clinical level it was recognized concurrently that outcomes of individual patient treatment programmes needed to be capable of measurement as to their success, i.e. to be evaluated.

Evaluation

This is the 'systematic process of determining the extent to which an action or set of actions were successful in the achievement of pre-determined objectives' (Hogarth, 1975). It is proving exceedingly difficult to apply this concept to evaluating physiotherapy practice. Three chief elements must first be defined in order to evaluate an individual patient treatment programme.

1. Pre-determined timed objectives (goal), e.g. this elderly lady will be able to walk 20 yards unaided by the end of two weeks.
2. The action or set of actions (input), e.g. daily physiotherapy (insufficiently specific), daily exercise on bed/plinth, balance and walking re-education (gives clearer picture of treatment programme). In a rigorous evaluation or research study it would be necessary to be even clearer than this regarding the exact details of treatment, including length and number of treatment sessions.
3. The extent of success (outcome). Methods for scoring outcome are notoriously difficult to devise, particularly if it is intended to use them consistently to evaluate the outcome of every treatment programme, e.g. At the end of treatment one of the following boxes can be ticked to indicate the result:

Symptom free (goal achieved) ☐   Much improved ☐
Slightly improved ☐   Same ☐
Worse ☐   Not known e.g. DNA ☐
(Clifton, 1984)

Although a valuable advance on 'patient much better' with its lack of objectivity, the above tabulation still has the following problems.

1. There is no meaningful numerical score.
2. 'Improvement' is still a subjective concept although for some very specific treatments outcomes can be objectively measured, e.g. joint range, muscle power.
3. Time taken/number of treatments/type of intervention (i.e. input) is not clarified.
4. It is difficult to define the outcome of a broad single goal.

Physiotherapists are currently struggling to create meaningful, useful, practical evaluation systems and in a number of departments have refined the above tabulation in various ways (see Chapter 3).

A broad single goal can be subdivided into sub-goals. At the end of treatment each sub-goal can be coded regarding the outcome of intervention:

1. Markedly worse
2. Slightly worse
3. Same/status quo/no progress
4. Slight improvement/progress
5. Marked improvement/progress
6. Goal achieved

This system creates a numerical score and breaks down a 'global' goal into sub-goals.

However, this whole endeavour is still beleaguered by a number of difficulties.

1. The need to differentiate between the patient's and the physiotherapist's perception of outcome and in some way incorporate them both.
2. The need to record in some usable way any other known factors external to the physiotherapy intervention which will have affected the outcome. (Unfortunately, many factors which affect treatment outcomes cannot be easily identified such as natural recovery or continuing degeneration.)
3. Any scoring system is vulnerable when the goal has not been fully achieved and the degree of improvement/progress must be scored. A classic example here is degree of relief of pain.
4. Physiotherapists, like many other health care professionals would rather treat patients than keep accurate, detailed treatment records!

Problem orientated medical recording (POMR)

Some of these difficulties can be overcome when this system is used. Systems vary in detail, but all have some common elements (see Chapter 1). POMR was originally developed as a total patient care medical record, with structured written input from all disciplines relating to a clearly defined list of an individual patient's problems. In practice, certainly in the UK, this system is rarely to be found in use even in specialist units, let alone general hospitals. If it were, it would have great advantages, in that patient care would become more orderly and comprehensive and thus prevent problems being overlooked or therapeutic effort being duplicated (see p. 19).

111

However, the problem-orientated approach can be used in writing physiotherapy notes even in the absence of an integrated multidisciplinary system. Clearly the above advantages of multidisciplinary use of POMR are not gained if the approach is only used by one profession. However, many other benefits accrue to the patient, the therapist and service provision/the profession. (The latter will be dealt with in the section on quality assurance.)

The advantages to the patient if the physiotherapist uses the problem-orientated approach are as follows:

1. The patient can be given a list of his problems (particularly in a rehabilitation unit) which enables him to be a more active participant in his rehabilitation.
2. The physiotherapist, having identified each physiotherapy problem of the patient, is more likely logically to pursue each problem.

There are also advantages for the physiotherapist:

1. Notes only have to be written when there are new or additional data.
2. There is clear ongoing documentary evidence as to whether or not the treatment is benefitting the patient. This enables the physiotherapist to evaluate treatment programmes and adapt them in response to progress (or lack of it) quickly.
3. Any physiotherapist, say one covering another's work, can easily identify what is wrong with the patient.
4. It is an effective means of self-evaluation and learning.
5. The physiotherapist's professional opinion can be clearly stated.

A problem orientated medical recording approach to keeping physiotherapy notes is becoming more commonly used in the UK.

Implementing a POMR recording system in a physiotherapy department is a major task, as the printed record sheets must be appropriate to the type of clinical work being carried out there. All physiotherapists need to be trained in a structured way. Having learnt how the components of the system link together and should be used, considerable discipline is necessary, particularly initially, to use the new format and not revert to the old ways of recording which were usually disorganized, incomplete, subject to whim and workload pressures. Differentiating between the various elements of the SOAP notes and slotting information in under the appropriate heading requires careful thought, and always remains to some extent arguable (Grieve, 1988).

112

Defining problems which are appropriate and sufficiently 'sized' to be amenable to physiotherapy intervention also requires skill and practice, e.g. 'inability to walk' may need to be broken into component problems for listing and clarifying initial plans and progress.

However, there is no doubt that using the POMR approach to physiotherapy record keeping provides a framework within which the outcome of clinical intervention with individual patients can begin to be evaluated using developing charting, scoring and measuring systems. These are increasingly reflecting both the patient's and the physiotherapist's perception of outcome, other factors external to physiotherapy which affected outcome and time taken/number of treatments or sessions/type of physiotherapy intervention made (e.g. teaching, advice, treatment).

Physiotherapists are also wrestling with the need to define problems so precisely that the outcome can be evaluated in terms of a yes/no answer, i.e. 'achieved' or 'not achieved', rather than subjectively trying to 'grade' improvement. In some systems, particularly those based on POMR, the outcome of intervention regarding *problems* is scored, in others the outcome vis-à-vis *goals* is measured. Measures or codes can be applied at discharge, or if goals/problems are precisely defined, for each treatment session, on a daily basis (Williams, 1986b, pp.11,16). This kind of system might be difficult to apply in certain specialties including possibly care of the elderly.

Evaluation is important not only for the individual physiotherapist working with the individual patient, but also for physiotherapy work with defined groups of patients. Individual physiotherapists should be more effective if they constantly monitor and evaluate the care they give their patients. However, unless they work with the peer group in their specialty actually to define an optimum standard of care, they and their managers remain vulnerable to questions about how 'good' their patient care is. In other words it is possible to measure outcome in the various ways discussed above, but unless an *overall standard* is set for expected performance as follows:

1. what percentage of goals should be achieved/what percentage of problems should be solved;
2. how much/what type of intervention should be needed;
3. how long the process of achieving goals/solving problems should take

the care an individual physiotherapist gives a patient cannot be objectively evaluated and performance level cannot be measured.

113

Retrospective patient care audit

This is a complex process which enables formal review of patient services to determine whether they achieved satisfactory results. It is introduced here and described later in this chapter (Ensuring effectiveness, p. 142).

It is significantly easier to review *outcome* than the *process* of care, i.e. the actions of the physiotherapist in assessing, treating, educating, advising etc., the patient. However, it is essential to review both in order to audit the quality of care. The source of data is completed POMR records for a specific, defined group of patients whose care is being reviewed.

It is clear that standardized POMR records must have been comprehensively completed if adequate data are to be extracted from them. However, in addition the relevant records must be extractable from the filing system. A number of identification methods can be used, depending on the type of physiotherapy service being offered. All have some inherent difficulties, but the most widely used system in physiotherapy is a standard classification of disease, e.g. ICD (International Classification of Diseases.) The classification number is entered on the record in an easily visible place and when an audit topic has been chosen the records of patients relevant to that topic are extracted.

An interesting common phenomenon in audit is that when routine practice is systematically studied, it is often found to differ considerably from what was assumed to occur (Shaw, 1980a).

Quality assurance

Some definitions of audit include the commitment to remedial action to correct deficiencies/improve care, others specifically exclude this aspect and are effectively only an assessment of quality. However, having evaluated the standard of care being given by a physiotherapy service to a defined group of patients, the logical next step is to take appropriate corrective action and then to re-audit in order to ensure that this aspect of patient care has in fact improved.

This latter process is one form of quality assurance which can be defined as:

A comprehensive concept which involves an *ongoing* programme of collection of data which is tested against predetermined *criteria* in order to *identify potential problems,* it further

114

involves a *commitment* and the *appropriate mechanisms* to use the information gained to *rectify the problems identified* and *improve the service* offered.

As can be seen, this comprehensive concept embraces both the concept of evaluation and quality assessment, but goes one step further in that it *ensures* quality according to predetermined criteria and standards. Various quality assurance models are in use, the one described below is the model developed by the American Nursing Association.

The steps in their quality assurance cycle are summarized in Table 7.1 and described here.

Table 7.1 Steps in quality assurance (ANA model)

1. Identify values, broad objectives - a philosophy of care

2. Identify/select appropriate:
   Criteria
   Standards
   Data collection tools

3. Collect data - continuously or sample

4. Interpret data and identify:
   Strengths
   Weaknesses
   Problems - potential, actual

5. Feedback data and identify possible courses of action

6. Choose from options and implement

7. Start again, i.e. cyclic process

Source: Quality Assurance in Priority Care Services, a discussion paper, Lewisham and North Southwark Health Authority.

1. *Identify values or broad objectives which essentially form a philosophy of care.* The process of 'teasing these out' can be quite lengthy and intellectually demanding, but the resulting statement forms the basis from which the rest of the process derives. The summary of key points in the Guidelines in Good Practice of the Association of Chartered Physiotherapists with a Special Interest in Elderly People (formerly ACPGM) are implied or actual values identified as being central in work with older people. They thus essentially form a philosophy of care:

   Key Point 1: Examination, assessment and recording
   Key Point 2: Co-operation with other team members

Key Point 3: Personal autonomy and personal responsibility for recovery

Key Point 4: Agreed goals, both short and long term

Key Point 5: Standards of physiotherapy and the importance of teaching

Key Point 6: Life-style – optimum levels of health and independence

Key Point 7: Evaluation

(These provide the topics for each chapter of this book although the order has been changed.)

2. *Identify/select appropriate criteria, standards and data collection tools.* An example of a *criterion* of quality which might be used is *interdisciplinary working.* Various aspects of interdisciplinary working could be used to assess its adequacy; one is the holding of regular case conferences. In order to evaluate this aspect, a *standard* needs to be set against which performance will be measured, e.g. the standard might be that case conferences are held weekly to discuss a particular group of patients. The *data collection tool* for this aspect might be a diary in which it was clearly recorded whether the case conference took place and whether the whole group of patients were reviewed.

This is a criterion which involves other professions, and this is true of many criteria which would be appropriate in quality assurance in the care of elderly people. In some respects this is clearly more difficult than a 'unidisciplinary' aspect would be, in that the co-operation of other professions must be gained.

An example of a 'unidisciplinary' *criterion* which might be chosen is *handover* of responsibility for mobility on discharge into the community from the physiotherapist to the patient, a carer, or another professional.

A *standard* must be defined for this and might be that on discharge of every patient into the community formal written handover will be carried out vis-à-vis defining the mobility goal and how to achieve it. The *data collection* tool for this might be a standard form which enables all staff clearly to record the required handover information. A copy of this must then be held in a standard place, e.g. the patient's physiotherapy record.

From these two examples it can be seen that criteria can be chosen for many different aspects of care. A framework covering all aspects of care comprehensively has been developed by

116

an American, Donabedian. This differentiates between *structure*, *process* and *outcome*.

(a) *Structure* is the setting in which care takes place.

(b) *Process* is what is done or the performance of care.

(c) *Outcome* is the result of care in terms of patient welfare or condition.

Each of these has its own tools, advantages and limitations. The ultimate aim is to demonstrate the linkage between them.

The example of multidisciplinary working discussed above fails within *structure*, whereas the aspect of handover is encompassed within *process*. *Outcome* is relatively self-explanatory although the most difficult of all to work on.

3. *Collect data.* This is done continuously or by a sample. The case conference example discussed above would probably best be studied by looking at each week in the diary, whereas the handover forms could be sampled, i.e. one in five of the discharged patients' records could be 'searched' to determine whether the handover form is there, and whether it is adequately completed.

4. *Interpret data and identify*
   (a) strengths
   (b) weaknesses
   (c) problems, potential or actual

5. *Feedback the interpreted data and identify possible courses of action.* This part of the process must involve the staff concerned, as they will only become really committed to whatever course of action is decided upon if they are involved in the discussion.

6. *Choose from options and implement.* All relevant staff whether uni- or multidisciplinary must also be involved in this stage of the process, in order for implementation to succeed.

7. *The cycle is recommenced.* An identical study may need to be undertaken again, or it might be modified, depending on the situation. Figure 7.1 shows a simplified quality assurance cycle.

Implementation of a quality assurance programme

In order to implement a quality assurance programme a quality assurance committee, usually consisting of multidisciplinary heads of services within an institution or facility must be set up. (This could develop quite easily from the traditional unit meetings attended by heads of department in a care of the elderly unit.) This

117

Figure 7.1 Cycle of quality assurance.

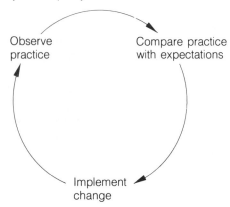

Source: Quality Assurance Project information leaflet, King's Fund Centre.

multidisciplinary committee would ensure overall quality of care.

Alternatively a committee could consist of all staff of one discipline working in a clinical specialty, e.g. all physiotherapists working with older people in a hospital. This would be similiar to a patient-care audit committee and would ensure quality of care in the specific service concerned.

The committee meets two, three, four or more times a year and carries out the steps identified in the ANA model above.

Recommended action is carried out by the appropriate managers through their staff, if a multidisciplinary headed service committee. If a specialist group of one discipline operating more on a 'peer' system, the action would be agreed and carried out by all the peer group. Although clearly, the more senior staff would be responsible for ensuring that the necessary action took place.

A full quality assurance programme requires considerable resources and therefore usually a long time scale for implementation. A simpler method of 'getting started' on quality assurance is to use the 'quality circles' approach.

Groups of staff (multi- or unidisciplinary) meet regularly, say every three or four weeks, and choose one specific item to concentrate on first, e.g. seating for older patients. Then they agree a realistic 'benchmark' standard, e.g. all older patients will be seated in a chair selected specifically for their needs within 2 days of arrival at the unit.

All staff are then bound to implement the agreed standard. Any problems in implementation are reported back to the quality circle

118

group which defines possible solutions and initiates action as considered most appropriate to solve each problem, e.g. difficulty in getting chairs portered from a store to the ward would need pursuing by the appropriate manager.

However, some problems may be insoluble and the standard may need lowering, e.g. 2 days to 3 days in the example used above. Alternatively the standard might be raised from 2 days to 1 day. When the seating item has been dealt with, i.e. a standard has been set and is being met, a decision is made as to when it will be reviewed. This might be for example in one to three months.

The quality circle group then goes on to choose a new item and pursue it as outlined above. Gradually the whole range of identified criteria under the headings of structure, process and outcome can be covered.

WHY ARE EVALUATION AND QUALITY ASSURANCE IMPORTANT?

Three main strands appear in answering this question. First, governments of developed countries are insisting that better health care must be provided at lower cost. Second, there is increasing pressure for accountability in health care. Finally, health care professions themselves, including physiotherapy, are becoming aware that they need to and need to be seen to be examining their work critically (Shaw, 1980b, p. 1509).

The need for accountability in health care

Consumers, both individually and in organized groups, are becoming much clearer about the health care service they want to meet their particular perceived needs. They frequently perceive their own needs differently from the way in which service providers identify them. There is an inherent tension in these two and sometimes opposing assessments of 'need' as the two 'sides' view the provision of health care from such different standpoints. Until recently this was all rather unstated and therefore undiscussed. However, consumers are now pushing the previously rather secretive medical professions into more open debate about service provision. Powerful individuals, consumer organizations and community health councils (consumer 'watch-dogs' appointed locally for each health district in the UK) are

119

in the forefront of this thrust and frequently have a very high local and national profile with concomitant press coverage.

Thus whereas traditionally, the need for health care by a particular patient or group of patients was determined by professional 'experts', the pendulum is definitely swinging in favour of a joint decision between the consumers and providers as to what is required. This clearly means some compromise between the 'demand' of the consumer and the more clinical definition of 'need' made by the provider which is always also coloured by an awareness of the limited resources available. Thus issues such as priorities, waiting-times, manner of reception, amount and type of treatment/intervention and results which can be anticipated, which are all about quality, are increasingly being debated and negotiated between the public and the providers of health care.

It is obvious that in order to be active in this difficult arena physiotherapists, like other professions have to be clear about what they are offering and about what it can be expected to achieve. To do this they must have evaluated their practice and be engaging in quality assurance. Interestingly the Royal Commission on the National Health Service (1979) recommended that hospital medical training posts should be approved only in departments where an 'acceptable method of evaluating care has been instituted'.

Quality is defined very differently by the following groups:

Customers
The general public
Providers of health care
Professional bodies
Management
Government

In any local or national debate regarding a particular health care issue the influence that each of the above can wield will vary and depend on their importance as a stakeholder in that specific debate.

The need to provide better health care at less cost

The Government insists that 'better' health care must be provided at less cost. Efficiency and effectiveness are the key concepts here.

Effectiveness has been defined as: 'The measure of the degree to which a particular treatment or pattern of care in the population

120

achieves its objectives in medical, psychological and social terms' (Long and Harrison, 1985).

It will be immediately recognized that this is a complementary definition to that given for evaluation above, i.e. effectiveness can only be determined by a process of evaluation; hence its importance.

However, the other side of this equation is *efficiency* which can be defined as: gaining maximum effectiveness (result) at least cost (minimum input).

The emphasis of all initiatives in the UK National Health Service over the last few years has been to gain ever-increasing effectiveness at ever-decreasing cost. This is necessary because the government is pledged to limit public-sector spending. In a climate where the costs of medical technology are rapidly increasing and there is a growing population of over-85-year-old people, who make big demands on health and social care resources, the challenge is to continue developing services to respond to changing needs, treatment possibilities and ideas of good practice on an effectively if not actually reducing budget (Maxwell *et al.*, 1983, p. 45).

Physiotherapy services must also respond to this challenge by being not only maximally effective, but also maximally efficient. A service which treats only a few patients extremely well (effective, but not efficient) is just as unacceptable as a similar one which treats large numbers of patients with poor clinical outcomes (efficiently but not effectively). This is represented in Figure 7.2.

Figure 7.2 Diagram illustrating relationship between efficiency and effectiveness.

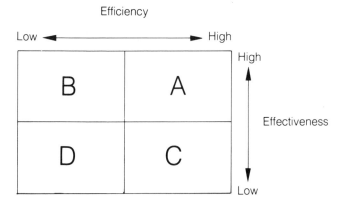

Source: Measuring efficiency in physiotherapy services, Occasional Paper No 3, Doncaster Health Authority Physiotherapy Service.

121

Any service in quadrant A is clearly successful in both efficiency and effectiveness. Services in quadrant B are clinically effective and therefore perhaps clinically acceptable, although inefficient. However, those in quadrants C and D are unacceptable due to clinical ineffectiveness and in the case of D additional inefficiency.

Figure 7.3 Efficiency model for physiotherapy services.

Resources

	Manpower	Facilities	Costs	Other resources	Income
5. District					
4. Hospital	QUESTIONS: AT EACH LEVEL				
3. Section	Is it effective to use the resource this way? Is this producing maximum results for least cost? Is it value for money?				
2. Individual physio.	What options have been considered and rejected as alternative uses of this resource? Was this resource used efficiently in terms of organization, planning, paperwork etc.?				
1. An individual intervention or treatment					

(left margin: Levels)

Source: Measuring efficiency in physiotherapy services, Occasional Paper No 3, Doncaster Health Authority Physiotherapy Service.

An exploration of efficiency in physiotherapy services at a national workshop in Doncaster (1986) led to the model in Figure 7.3. The resources available to physiotherapists can be grouped under the headings used in the model as follows:

Manpower   staff time, skill, knowledge and attitudes.

Facilities   departmental (including cost of heating, lighting, cleaning), other, e.g. ward, patient's home, residential home, day centre.

Other costs   ambulance and other transport, portering, telephone, post, library.

Other resources (people) nursing staff, social services staff (e.g. in

	residential homes), voluntary carers/ relatives, patients themselves!
Income	charity funds, course profits, private patients, rental of department (out of hours).

It is obvious that even small physiotherapy departments have significant resources available to them. Using them efficiently requires considerable managerial expertise at *every* level from the most junior newly qualified physiotherapist right up to district physiotherapist. Inexperienced physiotherapists, whose management responsibility is chiefly for their own time, need to concentrate particularly on time management so as to use this costly commodity as efficiently as possible. Using physiotherapy skills efficiently is inherent in the concept of delegation to and advising the people who constitute 'other resources', e.g. patients, relatives, care assistants, nurses. All physiotherapists need to be aware of 'marginal' costs. These are the costs incurred by carrying on treatment when it is not essential/necessary. The time used on these treatments/interventions could have been used for another patient needing essential treatment. Being able to discharge appropriately is an essential skill for every clinical physiotherapist. Prioritizing is another key skill, particularly for physiotherapists balancing heavy inpatient caseloads. It is vital to be able to determine which patients will not progress if they are not treated, and to know which patients will not regress if they are not treated. Opportunity costs are benefits lost when a choice is made to use resources in one way rather than another. Physiotherapists must apply this concept and think consciously about the benefit lost in progress of one patient if time is given to another (Williams, 1986c, p. 7).

Total caseload can be increased significantly (efficiency) without loss of effectiveness when physiotherapists vigorously question whether their use of resources is optimally efficient, i.e. whether they are producing maximum results for least cost. Only when the use of current resources can be proved to be maximally efficient and effective, can physiotherapists (or any other group) make a case for additional resources. It is, therefore, vital for physiotherapy services at all levels to be evaluated, so that physiotherapists can bid for resources to develop their services, which to the elderly are often very underdeveloped, particularly in the community. Even health districts which strictly have no development funds and are actively cutting services, will consider well-constructed cases for service development. These can of course be funded by the district using the concept of opportunity costs *across* services and maybe cutting a profligate service to fund a rigorously evaluated one which can justify expansion in line with district priorities. Having gained the funds, the challenge is to evaluate the performance of the new service from the outset against its objectives, so that it can be reviewed, found successful and its funding be ensured.

The Government not only sets the financial parameters within which services must now be provided, but also determines national policies for services. These are interpreted at regional and district level, but services provided to key groups within a unit of management in a local health district must be broadly 'in-line' with government policies and priorities. An example of this is the national policy regarding community care, this not only applies to mentally ill and mentally handicapped people, who are being moved from institutions back to their local communities but also to elderly people. It is now widely accepted that, in keeping with national policy, elderly people should if at all possible be enabled to remain in the community.

Local responsive community services must therefore be planned and provided which have as their objective keeping older people at home. In many districts the only way of gaining the finance to develop community services is to cut hospital services. This has largely been achieved by making them more efficient, often by cutting beds and increasing throughput. However, it is essential for the developing community services to be evaluated to ensure that they are fulfilling their aims and objectives. (As emphasized earlier these must be clearly stated so that performance can be measured.) Also the reducing hospital services must be reviewed to ensure that in the drive for greater efficiency, effectiveness is not sacrificed to an unacceptable degree.

The need for critical examination of practice

Against the above background it is clearly vitally important for individual health care professions to evaluate their practice and to go on to ensure the quality of their service. Physiotherapy being a young and therefore vulnerable profession has a particular need to do this. In fierce competition for resources, remedial therapy services are often seen as 'non-essential' by other groups. It can therefore be a matter of survival of services (and the profession) for physiotherapists to be able to 'prove' locally that they provide an effective and efficient service. Being a young profession not only means that it is less well-established in some clinical areas as an

124

essential service, but also that its body of knowledge is less well-developed. Proving the value of physiotherapy services has up till now relied largely on anecdote and subjective opinion. However, other tools are gradually becoming available to help with this predicament. They must however be *used* by clinical and managerial physiotherapists.

Research is gradually being published, which can be used locally to establish the value of a particular aspect of service. It is disappointing that many physiotherapists do not take note of sound research and adapt their practice accordingly. This makes them even more vulnerable to scrutiny and cuts. However, managers of physiotherapy services are increasingly aware of the need to ensure that their staff keep up to date with the literature and apply it in their clinical practice.

Evaluation, audit and quality assurance discussed above are all essential tools which enable physiotherapists to look critically at their work and to present factual cases to management locally as to the value of their work.

The measurement systems which have been used up till now in the NHS are not very useful in providing information which is meaningful regarding efficiency, effectiveness and quality. So-called national Performance Indicators for physiotherapy are currently only in-put indicators and make no attempt to measure clinical effectiveness or even activity, due to absence of usable data. Some other health service Performance Indicators do use *activity measures* such as bed turnover, in addition to input measures, but NHS indicators using the full four-stage model are still being developed (Table 7.2). The implementation of the Körner Steering Group on Health Services Information recommendations over the next few years will only provide limited measures of output in the UK. Even a well established, more comprehensive system such as that used in Canada is seen by many to have significant drawbacks.

There is therefore much work yet to be done in order to provide appropriate ongoing data, from which information can be extracted to enable physiotherapy managers to measure effectiveness and efficiency of their clinical services.

However, individual physiotherapists can, by rigorously using the concepts and tools of evaluation and quality assurance, ensure that an individual patient receives the most efficient and effective physiotherapy service possible. If all physiotherapists working with elderly people in a particular hospital, district or 'patch' (defined local geographical zone) work in this way the physiotherapy needs of the local population will be met as effectively and efficiently as

Table 7.2 Comparison of various models of quality assessment

	Aim/purpose	Input	Process	Output
Industrial model	To manufacture X items	Raw materials	Particular manufacturing process	Finished articles
Potential NHS performance indicator model	Objectives	Resources used	Activity measures	Outcome measures
Donabedian model	Philosophy/ aim	Structure	Process	Outcome/ result

possible. This increasing emphasis on providing a quality service in both the eyes of the consumer and the health care professional should, despite shortage of resources, increasingly satisfy the consumer and raise the satisfaction and morale of staff.

WHERE DO I BEGIN?

Working as a physiotherapist with older people is demanding and challenging. There is also usually an unlimited amount of work which could be undertaken. It is therefore essential to *'begin as I mean to continue'*, i.e. by working in an organized way, so as to provide a structure within which I can offer an evaluated, quality-assured service to my patients.

Job description

First, it is essential to have a written job description which provides the basis for understanding what is required of the physiotherapist in a particular job. It is impossible to tackle a job as complex as working with elderly people without a formal job description to define the parameters of the work. The job description will specify the grade of the post, accountability (this clearly states who the manager is to whom the physiotherapist is accountable) and responsibilities of the post. Some job descriptions first summarize the main areas of responsibility under headings e.g.

126

1. Assessment and treatment (clinical)
2. Liaison
3. Education and training
4. Management and administration
5. Health and safety

and then describe the detailed responsibilities under each of these headings. Although this creates a long job description it does make absolutely clear to a staff member what is expected and it thus also provides a useful baseline against which performance can be assessed.

Shorter job descriptions leave more to the imagination particularly of inexperienced staff and can lead to unstated expectations on the part of manager or staff member and therefore confusion in evaluating performance and doing the job. This is particularly true of work with elderly people where many subtleties are essential, e.g. knowledge of the home situation, liaison with carers regarding a joint approach to problems, ensuring that nursing staff know the mobility level at which a patient functions and how to encourage/enable performance at that level throughout 24 hours. For each member of staff to have a clear, accurate job description is considered to be an important aspect of the quality of service a health authority provides, as care and concern for staff is as important as that for patients.

Induction/setting objectives

It is also vital for staff to have discussed and agreed with the immediate manager objectives towards which to work. When starting a new job these will be quite short term and reviewed and revised frequently. They will initially allow new staff members adequate time to:

1. Read the departmental policies and procedures handbook;
2. Meet the staff with whom they will work, both of their own profession and others;
3. Take part in the best possible handover of patients/residents/clients from the previous physiotherapist to the new one.

This induction process is also a measure of the quality of management

127

in a workplace. It enables a new staff member to begin a job, not by 'picking-up' information haphazardly while meeting staff and patients in a rush at the same time as trying to take on a full clinical load, but by being able to absorb information gradually and create a personal framework within which gradually to take on the responsibility for clinical work. Even in a very busy department or service the time spent on accomplishing this induction even moderately well ensures that a new staff member can start off without falling immediately into a number of hurried inappropriate practices which run counter to provision of a quality service.

After induction, objectives are set which will be in the following areas:

1. Becoming familiar with departmental and hospital routines and practices;
2. Using the local record keeping system;
3. Becoming familiar with other key staff, patients and carers;
4. Becoming clinically active, gradually taking on a full work commitment.

Eventually objectives will be jointly set which focus on the areas with which the staff member is having difficulty, or wishes to gain expertise or development in and which reflect service needs.

Training needs

Many physiotherapists, when they begin to work with elderly people, have had no particular training in this very challenging field of physiotherapy. It is therefore important for the new staff member and manager together to determine whether the new recruit has the basic *knowledge*, *skills* and *attitudes* to function as a competent physiotherapist with this client group.

Clearly these exist at different levels, but if there are gaps in *basic* knowledge, skills and attitudes, *training needs* must be identified.

There are three main ways of fulfilling these training needs. *Courses* can be very valuable; they might be short, covering a very specific aspect of care, e.g. incontinence or motivation, or they might be longer embracing a whole range of topics. It is essential to ensure that the physiotherapist actually applies the knowledge, uses the skill or changes the attitude which the course was chosen to expand. This can be done by setting objectives and joint monitoring of progress on return from the course. *Study* of appropriate references, books and journals can be very helpful, particularly if the physiotherapist has the opportunity to discuss the subject concurrently with the peer group. Finally *visits* to other departments or units offering a similar service are often the most efficient way of 'boosting' skills, attitudes and even knowledge. Visits must be carefully arranged by the manager so that an appropriate programme is planned in advance to meet the needs of the visitor. Specific questions to be asked will need defining before the visit is made. Most important of all, the visitor will learn most from observing a committed, enthusiastic specialist physiotherapist in care-of-the-elderly in action and from subsequent discussion.

All these types of training will be more effective if the physiotherapist is required to give formal feedback to the rest of the 'home' department. A five-minute verbal presentation or relevant case presentation and ensuing discussion can be very successful in focusing on the key material which has been learnt.

Monitoring effectiveness

Having gained the basic knowledge, skills and attitudes to do the job, the physiotherapist must, in order to ensure quality in the work, focus very specifically on the needs of each individual patient. The data base must be thoroughly researched, the problem list accurately defined, plans and timed goals carefully determined and pertinent progress notes made. The whole process should be discussed with the patient at every stage and recorded systematically. The clinical work flowing from the assessment process must address the defined problems by working towards clear goals in a specified timescale. The achievement of goals must be continuously evaluated by the physiotherapist asking the question: 'am I/are we meeting these goals?'

For each physiotherapy intervention, i.e. every treatment or advice session, the physiotherapist must have a clearly defined objective in mind, which it is expected will be achieved in that time, e.g:

- during this session the patient will stand unsupported for 30 seconds;
- by the end of this session Mr X's wife will be able to transfer him unaided from wheelchair to bed;
- by the end of this home visit I will know if Mrs Y can manage her stairs unaided.

129

Each of these objectives has a yes/no answer regarding achievement which means that the physiotherapist can record the number of treatment sessions which achieved their objective and the number which did not (Williams, 1986b, p.16). These results can be discussed with the manager who will assess with the staff member whether too few are being achieved (in which case the goals may be set too 'high' or the clinical methods may be inadequate) or whether 'too many' are being reached (this may indicate that the goals are set too 'low'). The optimum achievement levels will need to be decided by manager and staff member and will certainly need to be monitored and reviewed. *Effectiveness* is thus being evaluated at individual clinical level by the physiotherapist and manager *jointly*.

Monitoring efficiency

The physiotherapist will also need continuously to monitor *efficiency* in respect of a number of aspects:

1. Planning the working day sensibly so that time is not wasted;
2. Ensuring that the number of patients seen and their outcomes are comparable with those of other staff of *the same grade and caseload*;
3. Prioritizing problems so that the work is usually contained within working hours. (If this is consistently impossible the manager and physiotherapist will need to determine whether the caseload is too high or being inefficiently handled.)
4. Using appropriate skills, both teaching and clinical, so that any physiotherapy intervention is capitalized on by patients and their carers;
5. Ceasing active treatment when optimum recovery has been gained and consolidated, ensuring that it is maintained by patient, carers and the environment (Williams, 1986c, pp. 12–13).

Record keeping

This vital activity is a key aspect of clinical practice in which 'good habits' must be maintained by each physiotherapist. So often records are seen as 'optional extras' which can be 'skipped', done 'after the patients have gone' or 'written at home'. The attitude which leads to this unprofessional behaviour was always both dangerous and

130

clinically unsound. It is now unacceptable in view of the need to assure quality in all aspects of patient care ('good' quality care cannot be given in the absence of adequate clinical recording), much-needed emphasis on evaluating patient care (which can only be done if records are adequate) and increasing litigation. Records must be kept accurately and fulfil legal as well as clinical and audit requirements. It is essential for the following information to be readily extractable for legal purposes.

Regarding a particular patient:

1. The dates on which he/she was treated by a physiotherapist;
2. What was done by the physiotherapist with or to the patient on each date;
3. Which physiotherapist treated the patient on each date.

In some POMR recording systems, each treatment and who gave it is not integral to the POMR record. This legally required information may therefore have to be specifically kept elsewhere or incorporated into the POMR record.

The format in Figure 7.4 can be used to audit records to ensure that they are adequately kept. Staff can use the checklist themselves and/or managers can sample records randomly using it.

Multidisciplinary working

Successful multidisciplinary working is crucial to providing quality health and social care services to older people. A new physiotherapist will thus need gradually to establish a place in the multidisciplinary team. This will be easier in a hospital unit where staff are all 'on-site' and are readily available for discussion. It should also be easier in a specialized care of the elderly or 'geriatric' unit, where the contribution of all disciplines is usually valued, than in a busy general medical or surgical ward setting where the role of therapists is often not fully understood or capitalized on. Multiprofessional work is particularly difficult in the community, where conscious thought must be given to arranging the necessary one-off joint-visits or case-conferences. Even getting to know the identity of the other professionals and carers who are working round a particular client can be difficult, although new multidisciplinary recording tools kept in the domiciliary setting are making this easier.

A key element of multidisciplinary work is an understanding of

131

Figure 7.4 Patient audit record.

Please tick appropriate box

Is the following information on the record: YES   NO   N/A

(a) Basic details about the patient:

    Record number

    Name

    Title

    Address

    Date of birth

    Telephone number — Home

                    — Office

    Transport details

    Occupation

    Hobbies

    Medical diagnosis

    Relevant medical history

    Relevant social history

    Status (I/P, O/P, P/P, Overseas visitor)

(b) Examination and treatment:

    Subjective data

    Objective data

    Problem list

    Short-term goals

    Timed goals

    Long-term goals

    Progress notes including treatment

    Response to treatment

YES   NO   N/A

Discharge summary related to:

— problem list

— short-term goals

— long-term goals

(c) Medical and surgical equipment:

Dates ordered

Dates delivered

(d) Administrative details related to therapy:

Source of referral

Date of referral

Review arrangements — medical

                    — physiotherapy

Record of involvement with other disciplines

Copies of correspondence

All entries dated

Name of therapist on record

Signature of therapist on record

Signature for each treatment

Source: Physiotherapy Services: A basis for the development of standards, King's Fund Centre.

each others' respective roles. Studies have shown that professionals usually have a distorted (often grossly) view of the roles of other professions. It is therefore essential for a physiotherapist gradually to clarify what she can realistically offer to the patients and the team. Expectations by other professions of physiotherapists will often be of 'treatment' in isolation from the carers and bearing no relationship to the patients' everyday life at home, in the ward or in a residential home. The physiotherapist has to work hard and long to convince, particularly the 24-hour carers, that physiotherapy with older people can only be effective if mobility and activity are seen as 'everyone's job', including the patients'. Physiotherapy treatment must be reinforced by the environment in which the patient lives; the appropriate chairs to ensure good seating positions, a bed of the correct height, the correct walking aid to hand and carers who have been shown by the physiotherapist how to handle an older person to achieve maximum functional mobility. Activity charts and entries in the multidisciplinary Kardex further reinforce this (see Chapters 4 and 5).

Formal multidisciplinary discussion about the goals and progress of particular patients is often organized to occur at case-conferences. The physiotherapist, along with other professionals, needs to attend these so that the problems which will be differently perceived by them all, can be jointly discussed. From this discussion, broad goals for each therapeutic discipline will be decided on and an overall goal and process agreed. Professional priorities will often vary and honest discussion and compromise is essential if the patient and relatives are not to be caught up in a maelstrom of confused or unfocused clinical activity (see Chapters 3 and 5).

Seeking information/knowledge

Finally, a physiotherapist newly appointed to a post working with older people, who wishes to work to a 'high' standard, needs to ensure his/her continuing education. It is essential always to ask appropriate, carefully phrased questions of senior staff of all disciplines when knowledge or skill is lacking. Similarly, honestly owning up that the answer to a received question is not known, is usually respected and avoids the confusion which surrounds a 'fudged' answer. Promising to go away and find out the answer usually satisfies the questioner, be he student, consultant, patient or relative. The library is an essential reference point. It is also vital to read the relevant professional journals and newspapers and to assimilate the contents and change clinical practice accordingly (i.e. stop doing things which don't work!). Physiotherapists are traditionally poor at this and cannot justify the use of the term 'professional' to describe them unless they genuinely keep up-to-date with knowledge, skills and attitudes.

HOW DO I CONTINUE?

Job and performance review

The thrusts for professional evaluation of clinical outcomes and greater accountability, efficiency and effectiveness in health care are also leading to a requirement for the performance of professional staff to be monitored and evaluated and for their work to some extent to be managerially controlled by their employer, be this the NHS or a private medical company. Limited resources must now be used to best effect to meet agreed objectives. Clinical practice which is known to be inefficient or ineffective must be replaced by practice which may not yet be rigorously researched but is widely recognized in the profession as being most appropriate. If this is not done in the NHS the nation's public funds are being wasted. Physiotherapy managers, along with managers of other health care professions, must now gradually guide, encourage and in the end specify what constitutes acceptable working practice, aware that pushing staff to change too hard or too fast may well have a negative effect. This process is incredibly difficult and is seen by some as an infringement of professional autonomy. In the end, however, 'he who pays the piper plays the tune' and all clinicians are now under considerable pressure to accept that they are accountable to the public via their employer for providing the highest quality service at least cost.

A staff development system is therefore needed wherein managers can work with staff to achieve the necessary changes of direction in clinical practice, attitude, or organization. Appraisal, which was often a one-way process with the manager telling the staff member how he was performing and not giving much guidance regarding how to improve, has been replaced in the NHS by Individual Performance Review (IPR). This model, initially for managerial levels, but now frequently used for all professional staff in a service is more of a two-way process. Very clear measurable personal and service objectives are set between the line manager and staff member, with agreed time scales for achievement and clearly defined tasks for

135

both to carry out, as managerial support and action is usually essential in order for a subordinate to achieve the required results. In addition when reviewing progress, the staff member is encouraged to point out difficulties which result from the way the job is structured or the style or actions of the manager. Thus progress is made by joint discussion, joint agreement of goals and tasks and joint performance review. This is not an easy process and appropriate training in listening skills, setting measurable objectives and monitoring is required by both the staff member and manager. The results, however, indicate that job satisfaction for both is increased and that for physiotherapists:

1. Time-management and making priorities are enhanced particularly for junior staff;
2. Problems are picked up *early* and appropriate timed plans are made jointly to address them;
3. Structured plans to enable all staff to develop clinically, managerially and personally are having the desired results.

For a new member of staff working in the complex area of care of the elderly in any setting, such a structured system is particularly valuable in providing on-going support with problems and development.

Self-monitoring and evaluation in isolation is extremely difficult, but within a structured system is enabled. Support is provided which encourages even the most junior therapist to pursue managerial, clinical and personal objectives. The threat inherent in 'one-way' appraisal systems is replaced in a 'two-way' job/performance review and staff development scheme by confidence that the needs of both the staff member and the organization can be met to a significant degree.

Control of workload; stress

Managers also have a very difficult additional responsibility to their staff and patients – the control of workload. This is particularly hard to do in an overloaded health care system. Achieving a balance between maximum efficiency/effectiveness and not overworking staff is becoming a major issue in assuring quality in health care. If staff are continually required to do too much they eventually suffer from 'burnout' and are unable to work effectively, sometimes for ever.

This in itself is inefficient as highly trained staff are lost to the service. The Brunel Institute of Organization and Social Studies found a few years ago, that workload of senior I physiotherapists was sometimes not well controlled by their superintendents (Ovretveit and Kinston, 1982). This is not surprising, as controlling workload is extremely demanding of managerial expertise and 'will'. The role of clinical therapists in ensuring that workloads are reasonable involves:

1. monitoring own workload
2. ensuring that own time management is optimal
3. ensuring that own priorities are made carefully with quality assurance built in, which may take *more* time
4. bringing unusual increase (or decrease!) in workload to manager's attention
5. in a positive way suggesting how the workload could be controlled (staff on the ground are often best-placed to do this)
6. at job and performance review formally discussing with the manager the implementation of workload control
7. recognizing own stress, i.e. when demands are beginning to outstrip personal coping resources
8. learning to manage own stress
9. using support of senior to help with all the above

It is salutory to discover that the very attributes which are looked for in potential physiotherapy students (enthusiasm, idealism and energy) are those which make a health care worker vulnerable to 'burnout'. This is because these 'desirable' traits often come with an inability to say 'no!' to work demands (Squires and Livesley, 1984), perfectionist tendencies and difficulty in compromising. Every clinician working with patients has, in the end, to make some sort of (often uneasy) peace with the notion that all the need can *never* be met – in my ward, my hospital, my district or nationally. Reaching this acceptance is usually traumatic, but unless it is reached, and boundaries are established around how much can reasonably be accomplished in a working day, physiotherapists and other health care workers face increasing stress and risk of 'burnout'. At junior level particularly, there may be a concern that not 'getting through' all the work is a sign of failure; there may be a solution to a problem causing this or it may be that there is just *too much* work. Managers must encourage their staff to talk openly about workload and stress.

137

Stress build-up depends on the interaction of many factors such as personality style (people with so-called 'Type A' personality are more liable to stress than 'Type B'), workload priority setting and quality demands, tension level in the individual or the department, and emotional state of the individual and other members of staff. Since stress is such an individual phenomenon, all staff need to be aware of the factors which increase their stress levels and also of their own personal signals of rising tension level. These can be:

1. wandering mind, faulty memory, increasing errors, less fluent speech
2. more frequent and noticeable tiredness, aching body, increasing irritability
3. mistakes, accidents, errors of judgement
4. decreasing humour
5. decreasing satisfaction in work and increasing desire to escape from work
6. eating, smoking, drinking increase

Stress can be more easily handled at work by staff member and manager if recognized early. Various stress-management techniques can then be built into the physiotherapist's working day and support given in ensuring that they are practised, e.g.

1. One or more periods of uninterruptible time must be allocated each day for listing, prioritizing and organizing tasks;
2. Timescales must be realistic and *one* task or problem at a time must be focused on in depth;
3. Set lunchtimes and finishing times are essential.

Other needs may be for an absorbing hobby, learning relaxation techniques or accepting personal limitations. Above all it is important for manager and staff member to recognize that there is a problem – potential or actual – to observe the pattern and to be prepared to make some commitment to change (Shaffer, 1982). This is an investment in quality for them and for the older patients who rely on them for care.

Improving service quality

Senior physiotherapists who have chosen the care of older people as their specialty will find that they gradually begin to address the

138

needs of identifiable groups of their patients, in addition to caring for their individual needs. A good example of this would be the realization that stroke sufferers and their relatives need considerable support both during the rehabilitation process and after active treatment has ceased. This realization might eventually lead to the establishment of a 'stroke group' to meet the identified need. A further example of this 'looking beyond' one-to-one direct clinical interaction to the broader needs of groups of patients would be the establishment of a regular *health education/promotion* group in a day hospital for elderly people. This provides a much-needed forum for discussion of how to keep active, prevent hypothermia, choose shoes and clothes, etc., and complements individual rehabilitation programmes. For many groups of patients the addition of educational/support programmes enhances quality of care by addressing health needs more comprehensively (Chapter 6).

These broader needs can be identified not only by professional staff but also by the consumers who surprisingly are rarely consulted about what their health care needs are. However, when they are consulted, really good ideas come forward and can be used in enhancing services, often making them more efficient and certainly more effective. The public is gradually taking more interest in and responsibility for its own health and health care professionals must capitalize on this. A measure of service quality is of course that both consumer *and* professional identify need and where possible work together to design 'packages' of care which will best meet that need.

Formal service review

Physiotherapists may identify ways of delivering more responsive services as a result of innovative thinking in the course of their usual clinical work and ideas may come forward from consumers, but in addition the effectiveness, efficiency and quality of services delivered to identified groups of patients should be *formally* reviewed from time to time. This is a necessary complement to the ongoing monitoring of outcomes of individual treatments and treatment programmes and consists on the one hand of formal peer clinical audit and on the other of looking at whether services can be provided in different ways to meet the needs of groups of patients. It may be discovered that clinical 'routines' have gradually and inadvertently become set for particular 'conditions' or groups. The care of the elderly specialty is especially vulnerable to this, as

139

progress can be very slow and patients may be 'on the books' for long periods of time, particularly in continuing care situations. This can lead to treatment routines which have long since ceased to meet patient needs being carried out, without review, by bored helpers or physiotherapists themselves. Examples of this might be:

- 'walking' continuing-care patients down the ward between two members of staff, when the patient is a less than active participant;
- indiscriminate use of apparatus, e.g. shoulder pulleys or small bicycle;
- 'exercise' classes in which too wide a range of patients is represented leading to a situation in which no one does any real exercise;
- repetitive exercise incorrectly done by bored patients, and targeted at no particular goal.

Clearly these aberrations should be discontinued and replaced by physiotherapy intervention which has a clear purpose in meeting the patients' needs. 'Walking' continuing-care patients might be replaced by joint work with nurses to establish individualized care plans which contain the means by which to maintain mobility; repetitive exercise with or without apparatus can be replaced by meaningful one-to-one or functional work; inappropriate exercise classes can be split up into smaller groups of similar ability for carefully chosen exercise or health education. It is important to recognize that 'routinization' of treatment can 'creep in' even in services which are considered to offer good quality. Even effective physiotherapy can sometimes be replaced by work which is more efficient, more enjoyable (for therapist or patient), more convenient, or in a more suitable location.

It is therefore essential for services to be regularly reviewed by all involved. Reviewing services under the headings in Table 7.3 has been found to be helpful. It is particularly important for current research findings to be known and applied when services are reviewed.

Once new staff have become established, managers should encourage them to look critically at the treatment methods or organization they may have inherited. This should avoid the situation in which a new physiotherapist 'takes over' a style of treatment without questioning it or feels that established ways should not be criticized.

140

Table 7.3 Service review - suggested aspects to be covered

1. Broad aim of service
2. Size of client groups (by condition or problem)
3. Objectives of service
4. How objectives are met
5. Current level of service
6. Handover
7. Problems
8. Review of relevant literature
9. Assessment of current service
10. Measures of quality assurance
11. Future needs
12. Recommendations

Ensuring efficiency

Aspects of work which need to be continually reviewed by established physiotherapists in addition to those listed on p. 130 are:

1. caseload handled
2. workload (broken down by percentage into clinical, teaching, management/administration)
3. number of treatments per case
4. appropriate allocation of work to physiotherapists on the basis of seniority
5. efficient timetabling
6. poor results are discussed and questioned informally (in addition to formal audit)
7. priorities are clear for when the staff complement is reduced due to absence
8. overall service objectives are set and achievement is monitored
   (Williams, 1986c, pp. 13–14).

A physiotherapist who becomes established in the care of the elderly specialty, will come to realize that teaching is a key element in the role. Efficiency and effectiveness must be considered when deciding whether to treat or teach a patient, or whether to teach the nurses, carers or relatives. The effectiveness of the teaching itself must be assessed, e.g. are the nurses now seating/handling patients correctly?

Achieving change

Changing situations which are considered unsatisfactory is always difficult. Sometimes an individual staff member working single-handed must tackle the problem alone, sometimes a team of physiotherapists can work together to achieve change. Either way, objectives for change must be set and the process for achieving them be agreed, both uni- and multidisciplinarily. The tasks individual therapists need to undertake within the overall process of change in order for the goal to be achieved must be agreed and incorporated within the job and performance review (appraisal) system. The achievement of all objectives must be measurable, both at individual therapist and 'team' level. The same principles should be used when commencing a new service.

Record keeping

The principles of good record keeping discussed must continue to be applied by physiotherapists as they become more experienced in any specialty, including care of the elderly (p. 130). Much of the monitoring of effectiveness and efficiency discussed here can only be carried out with adequate records.

Ensuring effectiveness

Many health care professionals who have been working in a specialized field for sometime begin to ask probing questions of themselves regarding their clinical practice. They may ask whether one treatment is more effective than another with a certain type of patient, whether a new treatment will achieve certain goals or whether the treatment they are giving is fulfilling the objectives set for a specific group of patients. The first two of these questions can only be answered by prospective clinical research. The third can be answered by carrying out *retrospective patient care audit*. The steps in this difficult but rewarding process are summarized in Figure 7.5 and outlined below. Staff interest in the audit and their participation in all these steps is essential:

1. Select audit topic – in physiotherapy audit this will usually be a treatment procedure or a diagnostic/clinical finding. The topic

Figure 7.5 The cycle of audit.

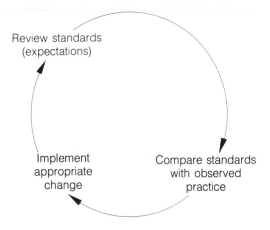

Source: Shaw, C.D. (1980b), p. 1444.

should be one which occurs frequently in the department and there should be some degree of consensus regarding its use for a particular kind of patient, e.g. stroke.

2. Select audit objective – the objective specifies the focus and should reflect the aspect of patient care within the audit topic that is most critical for successful patient treatment, e.g. to assess the ability to walk at the time of discharge from physiotherapy.

3. Draft audit criteria – this consists of developing a list of the specific indicators of care which are believed to be important. Each criterion must be able to be extracted from the records without the need for interpretation. Criteria must be relevant, measurable and achievable and must be understandable by all those who will extract data from the records. e.g.

   (a) Patient walks with or without assistance of one/walking aid on level surfaces inside.

   (b) Patient independent in standing from sitting and transferring from chair to bed.

   (c) Patient ascends and descends at least one step with handrail, with or without assistance of one.

4. Confirm criteria – this process must involve all those whose care will be reviewed and results in approval, modification or rejection of the draft criteria. In addition the anticipated level of performance for each criterion must be determined, e.g:

(a) Walking (as above) – 60%

(b) Standing from sitting/transferring (as above) – 90%

(c) Ascending/descending one step (as above) – 40%

Once an anticipated performance level is set the physiotherapists are committed to remedial action if the actual performance level is below the expected performance level. It can be imagined that the process of ratifying criteria can involve considerable negotiation, therefore the meeting (audit committee) at which this takes place must have clear ground rules and a person taking the role of arbitrator.

5. Extract data – from the physiotherapy records. This can be done by physiotherapists, helpers or clerks, but all must understand the criteria (which should be accompanied by agreed explanations) and must not interpret or judge the data retrieved. For each criterion and each record the appropriate one of the following possibilities is noted:

(a) present in the chart and criterion met

(b) present in the chart but criterion not met

(c) not present in the chart

Once all data have been extracted they are summarized in tabulated form.

6. Analyse data – the reconvened audit committee must determine from the above information whether their patient care is at, above or below the performance level agreed. In the case of the first two, no further action is necessary, however if performance level is below that agreed, the problem must be investigated. On reviewing the records which did not meet the criterion/did not include documentation regarding the criterion, valid reasons may be discovered for these discrepancies. These might include setting an unrealistic performance level and uncontrollable variables. However, if a 'true' performance deficiency has been identified, recommendations regarding appropriate corrective action must be made by the committee.

7. Corrective action – this will be taken on the basis of the importance of the deficiencies identified, e.g.

(a) gaps in skills/knowledge: continuing education/inservice training programmes

(b) management deficiencies (e.g. insufficient staff): controlling workload or drafting in more staff

(c) equipment deficiencies: make bid for additional equipment.

Responsibility and timescales for implementing agreed action must be clearly assigned. Checks should be periodically made to

144

determine whether the agreed action has been taken and appears to be successful.

8. Re-audit – the cycle is recommenced!

Multidisciplinary working

The principles of multidisciplinary working described in Chapter 5, continue, as with record keeping, to be an essential feature of the activity of physiotherapists working with older people. However, once a physiotherapist is well established in a multidisciplinary team, certain subtler aspects of this most sensitive constellation can be considered.

The difficult question of 'overlap' between physiotherapy and occupational therapy can be addressed and clarified. In order to *assure quality*, it is vital that responsibility for professional activity which falls in the 'overlap' area is clearly assigned in any working situation. Wheelchair assessment, certain activities of daily living, splint (orthosis) making and home assessment visits are areas which are often insufficiently clarified or even in dispute. Some of these tasks can be clearly allocated to one or other profession (e.g. wheelchair assessment, splint-making), others will need to be the subject of discussion and agreement vis-à-vis each client/patient (e.g. home assessment visits). Even in situations where there is too much work for all the combined therapist manpower to address, one or other profession may unreasonably try to annexe certain activities. This evidence of professional jealousy is unacceptable as it is wasteful of precious resources. The therapists concerned must, however painful, honestly discuss the issues and reach clear agreement which is adhered to and monitored jointly.

Further work can also be done on clarifying role expectations. Physiotherapists, particularly, need to work with care staff, nurses and relatives regarding agreeing a joint approach to handling and mobility. These need to be seen and accepted by others as the physiotherapist's key skills. The physiotherapist must complement this by seeing and accepting that these skills, to be useful, must be generously shared with all who handle and work with older people. There is no place for professional elitism.

In the current situation of seriously limited resources and growing concern about quality, there is great interest in the concept of *skills mix*. This focuses on the needs of the care group (e.g. patients in a day hospital, older disabled people living in the community) and

145

sets out accurately to define the proportional amount of input of different professional and non-professional skills (staff) necessary to fulfil these needs. It is clear that in many services, the numbers of staff of different kinds have grown (or not) as a result of a large number of factors other than client need, e.g. keen manager, recruitment drives. The availability of more data regarding clients and services is enabling general managers (those who manage comprehensive services to particular groups of patients in the NHS as per the recommendations in the Griffiths Report, 1981) to look at this question from an efficiency standpoint. Long-term shortages of professional staff and concern about wasteful overlap and unnecessary gaps in service on the one hand and insatiable needs of elderly and handicapped people worldwide on the other, pose a quality problem of enormous magnitude for managers of health care. Equipping all-purpose health care workers with the most basic skills of a variety of health professions in a short training period is seen as a possible solution. These workers, who are appearing in all parts of the world, may be called generic health care workers, support workers, multi-therapists or therapy aides. In the UK the National Audit Commission recommended the creation of a new occupation called 'community carers'; Sir Roy Griffiths in the recent report Community Care: Agenda for action (1988) supported this development.

There are situations in which work can be carried out more efficiently and effectively and to a higher standard if resources of all kinds are shared by professional groups. A remedial helper who does activities of a physiotherapy *and* occupational therapy nature can be a better use of resources in some situations than a helper who only does one or the other. Some group activities can be best done by staff of a variety of disciplines, e.g. groups practising functional activities.

Continuing education

This vital topic was introduced at the appropriate level for the newly appointed physiotherapist (pp. 128 and 134). Here it is expanded for the more experienced physiotherapist who is gradually deepening and broadening skills, knowledge and attitudes in a specialty.

Physiotherapists working with older people need to become expert clinicians in situations of multiple pathology and problems, but they also need to be skilled teachers. In a survey asking older people what they most wanted their physiotherapist to be, 'a teacher' was the

146

most frequent answer. (Whereas the physiotherapists working with older patients thought being 'kind, friendly and caring' most important.) They also need to have an armoury of counselling and communication skills to draw on in the many situations with patients and relatives where clinical skill can only be useful once certain other matters like expectation about progress/prognosis, motivation and loss have been explored. Consequently the need for further training is usually in these areas of broader skill which are not specific to physiotherapy, whereas learning how to prioritize a patient's multiple problems is usually the result of sheer volume of experience. Knowing who to refer patients on to, when emotional/ psychological or other problems are too complex or difficult for a physiotherapist to address in the context of her essentially rehabilitative role, is also important and develops as these problems are gradually recognized and the appropriate services to deal with them identified.

Visits to and seminars with peers doing similar work, which give the opportunity for discussion and preferably structured debate, will become more important than purely clinical courses, although these too will have their place. Projects are another very helpful way of studying a chosen aspect of the care of elderly people in more detail, and can have valuable additional results in identifying necessary change. Role development and management courses will sharpen a clinician's eye to issues of the most efficient and effective use of resources and will help to provide strategies for taking action to achieve necessary change. Membership of the Association of Chartered Physiotherapists with a Special Interest in Elderly People provides a national peer group with whom to compare practice, and develop policies and standards.

Many of these aspects of continuing education are important for physiotherapists on rotation schemes in the specialty as well as for those who will remain in it.

Finally, it is worth reiterating the point regarding staying up-to-date with the literature, not only journals for physiotherapists, but also appropriate medical and social services publications.

Throughout, this and other sections it has been assumed that a manager is available to work with the physiotherapist on job and performance review, objective setting and identifying/meeting needs for continuing education and development. However, it is recognized that this support is not always available, in which case peer support and peer review become even more important. Ultimately, however, an isolated physiotherapist working alone in this demanding specialty must become an expert in self-monitoring, self-criticism and self-directed learning.

HOW ARE EVALUATION AND QUALITY ASSURANCE DIFFERENT WITH OLDER PEOPLE?

Evaluation – difficulties

Variables

It is widely acknowledged that evaluating the effectiveness of physiotherapy is extremely difficult. This is due to the large number of variables which operate, even when physiotherapy is the only therapeutic intervention a particular patient is receiving. The process of physiotherapy is essentially dynamic and involves the physiotherapist using a variety of techniques, approaches and educational strategies at different stages of a treatment programme or within one treatment session; a 'standardized treatment' which makes evaluation reputedly easier will usually be unrealistic and research using such a notion is usually unhelpful. The patient too will react individually to the treatment, the condition and the therapist. Cecily Partridge explores these issues in an important article (1980) and goes on to suggest a classification which groups together patients who have conditions with similar features and where the outcome of physiotherapy intervention can be considered in a similar way. There are four groups in this classification which is introduced in Chapter 3, p. 45.

It is clear that the complexity of evaluating the effectiveness of physiotherapy increases progressively from group 1 through to group 4. It is easier to evaluate a treatment which can be hoped to effect a 'cure' and usually involves only the physiotherapist and patient, than one which concentrates more on achieving and maintaining function and often involves a number of different carers.

Multipathology

Evaluating the effect of physiotherapy with older people is even more complex, because they usually, particularly in the 'very old' age group which is increasingly represented in physiotherapists' caseloads, suffer from conditions in two or more of the classified groups at the same time. This multiple pathology poses enough

148

difficulties for the practising clinician; for the physiotherapist who wishes to evaluate or research treatment outcomes it greatly complicates an already difficult process.

Multiple involvement

Not only are multiple problems present but, in addition, a variety of other therapeutic interventions are often taking place, e.g. drug regimes, occupational therapy, nursing procedures. Factors which operate for younger people may also complicate researching physiotherapy with older patients, e.g. complicating conditions such as mental health problems, co-operation with the therapist and compliance in carrying out instructions in between treatment sessions.

However, some physiotherapists are engaging with this challenging work and much groundwork can be done in small local studies. So called 'pure prospective research' is necessary so that the value of physiotherapy can be scientifically proved or disproved, but 'action research' which is more descriptive and less comparative and 'participation research' which involves clients and the community can be useful and are less demanding of research skill, time and finance. Physiotherapists who decide not to become involved in research can contribute much by retrospectively auditing their practice as described earlier.

Quality assurance issues

Keeping up-to-date with advances in gerontological knowledge

In order to set criteria and deliver services of high quality all physiotherapists working with older people need to recognize the great advances which are being made in the knowledge of many aspects of ageing. For some years this area of enquiry languished behind others but it is now receiving more attention and funding. The biology of ageing now recognizes that ageing carries with it a decrease in the functional capacity of all body systems, the rate varying with the individual. The effect of ageing on all these systems is being studied. It is necessary for physiotherapists to keep up-to-date with new knowledge of the systems particularly relevant to them, so that they can adapt their practice accordingly. For instance, it has now been *proved* that there is a significant relationship between physical inactivity and a decline in mental function. Physiotherapists

149

have long suspected this, but can now draw on scientific certainties when convincing carers how important it is to keep older people mobile.

Gerontological studies are being carried out worldwide on sociological and psychological aspects of ageing. Physiotherapists need to draw on this so that they can understand the difficult process an individual must adapt to during the passage between adulthood and death. Psychological traumas such as bereavement, loss (e.g. of role, independence, home, choice, control of environment) frustration, loneliness and loss of predictability, can at least temporarily seriously affect an older person's ability to cope with illness or disability and a holistic approach to the patient can only be maintained through understanding of these emotional difficulties (Chapter 2). Sociologically, older people often have to live on a reduced income, have lower status in the community and often live in inadequate housing. These factors adversely affect their health and their well-being and need to be alleviated as much as possible by calling on the appropriate services and community support in order for any physiotherapy programme to have a reasonable chance of success. Even where deprivation and other social problems cannot be significantly alleviated, an understanding of them will help a physiotherapist in setting realistic standards for rehabilitation work with older people in the community or in hospital. Issues which frequently arise are the necessity/advisability of moving into sheltered housing or residential accommodation and the whole question of discharge from hospital, which revolves around so many complexities including psychological and sociological factors. Knowledge of these would be essential in any quality assurance programme to ensure the optimum discharge practice.

Geriatric medicine, too, is fast increasing its body of knowledge and skills. Physiotherapists working with older people will need to 'keep up' with these developments in terms of drug usage and other medical advances. New surgical techniques, particularly orthopaedic, must be understood in order for continuing rehabilitation programmes to be relevant and realistic. Developments across the spectrum of medicine, both conventional and alternative will often have a bearing on work with older people, so need to be kept in touch with.

Since physiotherapists usually work within the 'medical model', advances in medicine are usually absorbed in the course of daily work, however knowledge of growth in gerontological, sociological, psychological and biological knowledge must often be specifically pursued and is a professional responsibility despite the acknowledged difficulties in access.

Demanding nature of the work

Despite the fact that care of the elderly is the longest established specialty within the priority care areas of physiotherapy, it is still proving difficult to attract physiotherapists to work in this fascinating field. This sometimes results in unfilled posts at senior level and junior staff rotating for a few months into the specialty with minimal supervision and training, or it can result in dedicated senior staff working with insufficient junior staff where rotation schemes have not been established. Whatever the situation, care of the elderly units often have limited physiotherapy manpower which results in a potential amount of work which exceeds the resources available to deal with it. It is essential for senior physiotherapy managers to define with the staff working 'on the ground' the amount and type of work which can realistically be done with limited resources. This process is essential in order to safeguard service quality. Despite the difficulty in saying 'no' to medical staff, patients and relatives it is sound professional practice to limit work to that which can reasonably be done well, rather than to succumb to unrealistic demands and carry out work of poor quality which lowers staff morale and does little for patient care.

Not only do physiotherapists working with older people usually work very hard in order to respond to the multiple needs of their patients/clients, but they also get little direct feedback from them. Older people needing physiotherapy are usually struggling to cope with a number of adverse circumstances, of which regaining mobility is not always the first priority. Therefore, at worst, they may feel the physiotherapist is just another problem and wish they could be left in peace. This clearly leads to the physiotherapist having to work hard to overcome the resistance, with little chance of a 'thank you'. At best, patients may co-operate very positively with the physiotherapist who makes them uncomfortable, exhorts them to move when it is an extreme and painful effort and almost always has another goal waiting to be tackled as soon as the previous one has been mastered. Even well-motivated patients are often very stressed by their illness or disability and the life events surrounding it and have little spare personal resource to be very grateful to their energetic physiotherapist.

Physiotherapists must recognize that lack of verbal feedback is a deprivation in this work but try not to allow it to affect the quality. In addition progress is often extremely slow, which requires immense patience and persistence. All this at times leaves the physiotherapist drained. The difficulties and demands of this work must be acknowledged and the tactics to avoid burnout mentioned earlier are vitally important for quality to be assured for patients and staff. It is self evident that this area of physiotherapy must be approached within an 'enabling/caring' model not a 'curing one'.

Responsibility for mobility in the community

Many, perhaps most, physiotherapists in this field work in hospitals. It is vital for them to work closely with their few community counterparts to provide a seamless service for patients who are discharged from hospital and need to be followed up in the community. With patterns of increasingly early discharge, limited community resources need to be very carefully used. Close and accurate communication between the two groups of physiotherapists is necessary so that no resource is wasted – neither the intensive hospital rehabilitation which can be lost through insufficient follow-up, nor the community physiotherapy which can be wasted if used routinely, without careful thought.

Handover of responsibility for a patient's mobility, either to be maintained or gained further, can also be made to other health or social services staff, volunteers/friends or the patient's relatives. Physiotherapists, as the professional custodians of mobility, must not take their duty to hand over this responsibility for mobility lightly. This may consist of discussing with husband and wife together how he should mobilize, e.g. she might serve all meals and snacks in a different room to the one her husband spends the day in so that he, although disinclined to be active, has several short walks each day. A care-assistant in an old people's home may need to be shown (or informed) how to encourage and minimally to assist an elderly lady to walk with a frame as she becomes more mobile following a repaired fractured neck of femur. A home help may need to be informed of the independence level at which a client should carry out functional activities like getting out of a chair, walking and managing stairs. If the client's performance deteriorates the home help should have the physiotherapists' telephone number to call for assistance. All this constitutes good practice, but the patient should also have a role in being given some responsibility for maintaining mobility which has been gained through such toil and through the use of such an expensive resource as physiotherapy. Involvement of the old person in the rehabilitation process as an active partner from the beginning might make this a process more commonly and successfully carried out than at present. Old people are still seen, even by some specialists in the field, as incapable of active participation in their care. This is true of probably only a small minority of patients, but is a continuing reflection not only of physiotherapists' attitudes, but also of those of other workers and society in general.

Expectations of activity in older people

Older people are vulnerable and it is very difficult to strike a balance between sensitive care which enables them to make their own decisions in their own time, even if the result involves some appropriate risk-taking, on the one hand and neglect of an old person who is in a situation of unacceptable risk in the community, on the other. A similar issue is of great concern to the physiotherapist: the fact that most people in society, including the elderly themselves, have very low expectations of their health, fitness and activity levels. Thus it is usually accepted that older people will become gradually immobile as though ageing were itself a disease. The confusion here is between the greater prevalence of several disabling diseases in old age and the ageing process itself, which as many fit, active older people constantly prove does not *ipso facto* lead to immobility. Physiotherapists working with older people have a unique role in clarifying this fact with as many people who they come into contact with, all of whom will themselves one day become older people.

Engendering a positive attitude towards elderly people and their potential in all possible contexts and settings is long-term quality assurance work and it forms an important component of the increasing lobby which upholds the rights and needs of ageing people.

Acknowledgements

Thanks are due to Patricia Burke and Joan Roberson who gave valuable help in the preparation of this chapter.

References

Abrams, M. (1978) *Beyond Three Score and Ten*, Age Concern.

ACPSIEP (1985) Physiotherapy with Elderly Patients; Guidelines in Good Practice, p. 3.

Adler, S. (1985) Self care in the management of the degenerative knee joint. *Physiotherapy*, **71**, 58–60.

Argyle, M., Jestice, S. and Brooks, C. (1985) Psychogeriatric patients – their supporters' problems. *Age and Ageing*, **14**, 355–60.

Ayalon, J., Simkin, A., Leichter, I, and Raifmann, S. (1987) Dynamic bone loading exercises for post menopausal women. *Archives of Physical Medicine and Rehabilitation*, **68**, 280–3.

Birren, J. and Woods, A. (1985) Psychology of ageing, in *Principles and Practice of Geriatric Medicine* (ed. M.S.J. Pathy) Wiley, Chichester.

Bohman, I. (1987) The Bobath approach and the geriatric stroke patient. *Clinics in Physical Therapy*, **14**, 183–95.

Brooks, D. (1986) Teams for tomorrow – towards a new primary care system. *Journal of the Royal College of General Practitioners*, **36**, 285–6.

Brown, R. and Frith, C. (1986) Some psychological factors relevant to physiotherapy in patients with Parkinson's disease. *Physiotherapy*, **72**, 335–7.

Caird, T. and Judge, T. (1979) *Assessment of the Elderly Patient*. 2nd edn, Pitman Medical, London.

Chartered Society of Physiotherapy (1986) Rules of professional conduct. *Physiotherapy*, **72**, (Suppl.).

Clarke, M., Lowry, R. and Clarke, S. (1986) Cognitive impairment in the elderly – a community survey. *Age and Ageing*, **15**, 278–84.

Clifton, S. (1984) Manipulating Physiotherapy, *Health and Social Service Journal*, 19 April, p. 467.

Clough, R. (1981) *Old Age Homes*. Allen & Unwin, London.

Cole, G. (1985) Neuropathology, in *Principles and Practice of Geriatric Medicine* (ed. M.S.J. Pathy) Wiley, Chichester.

Cullinan, T. (1986) *Visual Disability in the Elderly*. Croom Helm, London.

Davis, C. (1986) The role of the physical and occupational therapist in caring for the victims of Alzheimer's disease, in *Therapeutic Interventions for the Person with Dementia* (ed. E.D. Taira), Haworth Press

Documentation and Retrieval Group of the Chartered Society of Physiotherapy (1988) *Record Keeping*. Kings Fund Centre, London

Ellis, M. and Munton, J. (1982) *Are you sitting comfortably? A guide to choosing easy chairs*. Arthritis and Rheumatism Council from PhD Thesis 'Forces in the human knee when rising from a chair'.

Fansler, C., Poff, C. and Shephard, K. (1985) Effects of mental practice on balance in elderly women. *Physical Therapy*, **65**, 1332–6.

Fernandez, S. (1987) Physiotherapy prevention and treatment of pressure sores. *Physiotherapy*, **73**, 450–4.

Finlay, O., Bayles, T.B., Rosen, C. and Milling, J. (1983) The effects of chair design and cognitive status on mobility. *Age and Ageing*, **12**, 329–35.

Finn, A.M. (1986) Attitudes of physiotherapists towards geriatric care. *Physiotherapy*, **72**, 129–31.

French, S. (1988) History taking in the physiotherapy assessment. *Physiotherapy*. **74**, 158–60.

Grieve, G. (1980) *Common Vertebral Problems*, Churchill Livingstone, Edinburgh, p.169.

Grieve, G.P. (1988) Clinical examination and the soap mnemonic, *Physiotherapy*, **74**, 97.

Griffiths, R. (1983) NHS management enquiry: Recommendations for Action, DHSS. (Griffiths Report, 1981).

Griffiths, R. (1988) *Community Care: Agenda for Action*, HMSO, London, pp. 25–26.

Hare, M. (1985) The physical problems of depressive illness. *Physiotherapy*, **71**, 258–61.

Hare, M. (1986) *Physiotherapy in Psychiatry*, Heinemann Medical, London.

Hargreaves, S. (1987) The relevance of non-verbal skills in physiotherapy. *Physiotherapy*, **73**, 685–8.

Hawker, M. (1975) Motivation in old age, the physiotherapist's view. *Physiotherapy*, **61**, 182–4.

Hesse, K. and Campion, E. (1983) Motivating the geriatric patient for rehabilitation. *Journal of the American Geriatric Society*, **31**, 586–9.

Holden, U. and Woods, R. (1982) *Reality Orientation*. Churchill Livingstone, Edinburgh.

Ice, R. (1985) Long term compliance. *Physical Therapy*, **65**, 1832–9.

Isaacs, B. (1985) Clinical and laboratory studies of falls in old people, in *Clinics in Geriatric Medicine*, (eds T. S. Radebaugh, E. Hadley and R. Suzman), Vol. 1 No. 3, Falls in the Elderly: Biologic and Behavioral Aspects, W.B. Saunders, Philadelphia.

Isaacs, B. and Akhtar, A.J. (1972) The set test – a rapid test of mental function in old people. *Age and Ageing*. **1**, 222–6.

Lawler, H. (1988) The physiotherapist as counsellor, in *Physiotherapy in the Community*, (ed. A. Gibson), Woodhead Faulkner.

Ley, P. (1972) Primacy, rated importance recall of medical statements. *Journal of Health and Social Behaviour*, **13**, 311–17.

Long, A.F. and Harrison, S. (1985) *Health Services Performance Effectiveness and Efficiency*. Croom Helm, London, 12.

Macdonald, J. (1985) The role of drugs in falls in the elderly, in *Clinics in Geriatric Medicine*. (eds. T.S. Radebaugh, E. Hadley and R. Suzman), Vol. 1 No. 33, Falls in the Elderly: Biologic and Behavioral Aspects, W.B. Saunders, Philadelphia.

Maitland, G. (1977) *Peripheral Manipulation*. Butterworths, London.

Maxwell, R., Hardie, R., Rendall, M., Day, M., Lawrence, H., Walton, N. (1983) Seeking quality, *Lancet*, **i**, 45–8.

Overstall, P., Johnson, A.L. and Exton Smith, A.N. (1978) Instability and falls in the elderly. *Age and Ageing*, **7**, (suppl.), 92–6.

Ovretveit, J. and Kinston, W. (1982) Unpublished report Regional Workshops on Organisational Problems in High Level Clinical Physiotherapy (for CPS steering committee).

155

Partridge, C. (1980) The effectiveness of physiotherapy – a classification for evaluation, *Physiotherapy*, **66**, 153–5.

Partridge, C. (1984) Recovery from conditions involving physical disability. *Physiotherapy*, **70**, 233–5.

Pentland, B., Pitcairn, T., Gray, J. and Riddle, W. (1987) The effects of reduced expression in Parkinson's disease on impression formation by health professionals. *Clinical Rehabilitation*, **1**, 307–13.

Pratt, J.W. (1978) A psychological view of the physiotherapist's role. *Physiotherapy*, **64**, 241–2.

Primary Health Care – a review (1976) HMSO, London.

Pritchard, P. (1981) *Manual of Primary Health Care: Its Nature and Organisation*. 2nd edn, Oxford University Press, Oxford.

Pritchard, P. (1984) How can we improve team working in primary care? *The Practitioner*, **228**, 1135–9.

Purtilo, R. (1984) Applying the principles of informed consent to patient care, *Physical Therapy*, **64**, 934–7.

Ransome, H. (1980) The role of the physiotherapist in homes for the elderly. *Physiotherapy*, **66**, 324–31.

Richie, C. and Lough, J. (1988) The Ritchie–Lough Charting System, *Physiotherapy*, **74**, 274.

Royal Commission on the National Health Service (1979) Measuring and controlling quality, in *Report of The Royal Commission*, pp. 173–7.

Shaffer, M. (1982) *Life After Stress*, Plenum Press, New York.

Sharon, D., Kritek, B., Shaver, B., Blood, H. and Shephard, K. (1986) Age bias: physical therapists and older patients, *Journal of Gerontology*, **41**, 706–9.

Shaw, C.D. (1980a) Aspects of audit; 2 Audit in British Hospitals, *British Medical Journal*, 31 May, 1314–16.

Shaw, C.D. (1980b) Aspects of audit; 4 Acceptability of audit, *British Medical Journal*, 14 June, 1443–6.

Shaw, C.D. (1980c) Aspects of audit; 5 Looking forward to audit, *British Medical Journal*, 21 June, 1509–11.

Shephard, A., Blannin, J. and Smart, M. (1980) The role of the nurse, in *Incontinence and its Management*, (ed. D. Mandelstam) Croom Helm, London.

Shephard, R.J. (1985) Physical Fitness, in *Principles and Practice of Geriatric Medicine* (ed. M.S.J. Pathy), Wiley, Chichester.

Simek, T. and O'Brien, R. (1978) Immediate auditory feed-back to improve putting quickly. *Perceptual and Motor Skills*, **14**, 1133–4.

Sims, J. (1983) Ethical considerations in physiotherapy, *Physiotherapy*, **69**, 119–20.

Spragg, A.K. (1984) *Psychological problems of caring*, Alzheimer's Disease Society, London.

Squires, A. and Livesley, B. (1984) Beware of burnout. *Physiotherapy*, **70**, 235–8.

Squires, A.M. and Simpson, J.M. (1987) The impact of clinical experience in geriatric medicine on physiotherapy students. *Physiotherapy*, **73**, 516–21.

Steffen, T. and Meyer, A. (1985) Physical therapists' notes and outcomes of physical therapy, *Physical Therapy*. **65**, 213–17.

Stewart, M.C. (1980) Incontinence and the team in geriatric medicine, in *Incontinence and its Management* (ed. D. Mandelstam), Croom Helm, London.

Thompson, M.K. (1980) Management of the elderly patient in the community, in *Incontinence and its Management* (ed. D. Mandelstam), Croom Helm, London.

Vandervoort, A., Hayes, K. and Belanger, A. (1986) Strength and endurance of skeletal muscle in the elderly. *Physiotherapy Canada*, **38**, 167–73.

Vellas, B. and Cayla, F. (1987) Prospective study of restriction of activity in old people after falls, *Age and Ageing*, **16**, 189–93.

Wagstaff, G. (1982) A small dose of common sense – communication, persuasion and physiotherapy. *Physiotherapy*, **68**, 327–9.

Warnock, M. (1983) *The Nature of Choice*, Occasional paper 8, Age Concern.

Wattis, J. and Church, M. (1986) *Practical Psychiatry of Old Age*, Croom Helm, London.

Williams, J.I. (1986a) Physiotherapy is handling. *Physiotherapy*, **22**, 66–70.

Williams, J.I. (1986b) *Monitoring Effectiveness in Physiotherapy Services*, Occasional Paper No. 2, Doncaster Health Authority, Physiotherapy Service.

Williams, J.I. (1986c) *Measuring Efficiency in Physiotherapy Services*, Occasional Paper No. 3, Doncaster Health Authority, Physiotherapy Service.

Williamson, J. (1981) Screening, surveillance and case finding, in *Health Care of the Elderly* (ed. T. Arie), Croom Helm, London.

Williamson, J., Smith, R.G., Burley, L.E., (1987) *Primary Care of the Elderly*, Wright, Bristol.

Yesavage, J.A., Brink, T.L. (1983) Development and validation of a geriatric depression screening scale, *Journal of Psychiatric Research*, **17**, 37–49.

Further reading

General information

Blyth, R. (1979) *A View in Winter*. Allen Lane, London.

Carver, V. and Liddiard, P. (eds) (1978) *An Ageing Population*. Hodder & Stoughton with the Open University Press, Sevenoaks.

Documentation and Retrieval Group of the Chartered Society of Physiotherapy (1988) Record Keeping, King's Fund Centre, London.

Personal care and advice to carers

Caring for the Person with Dementia (1984) Alzheimer's Disease Society, Bank Buildings, Fulham Broadway, London SW6 1EP.

Franklyn, S., Perry, A. and Beattie, A. (1982) *Living with Parkinson's Disease*. Parkinson's Disease Society, 36 Portland Place, London W1N 3DG.

Fry, J. (ed.) (1980) *Primary Care*. William Heinemann Medical Books, London.

Gore, I. (1979) *Age and Vitality*, Unwin, London.

Help at Hand. The Who, How, Where of Caring. Association of Carers, Medway Homes, Balfour Road, Rochester, Kent.

Henley, A. (1982–4) *Asians in Britain*, 3 vols. *Caring for Sikhs and their Families*; *Caring for Muslims and their Families*; *Caring for Hindus and their Families*. DHSS and King Edward Hospital Fund for London.

Hodgkinson, J. (1988) *Homework: Meeting the Needs of Elderly People in Residential Homes, Booklet No 3, Promoting Mobility*. Centre for Policy on Ageing, 25–31, Ironmonger Row, London.

Parkes, C.M. (1975) *Bereavement Studies of Grief in Adult Life*. Penguin, Harmondsworth.

Index